MacLeod's Introduction to Medicine

Jonathan Waxman

MacLeod's Introduction to Medicine

A Doctor's Memoir

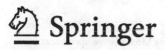 Springer

Jonathan Waxman
Faculty of Medicine
Imperial College London
London
United Kingdom

ISBN 978-1-4471-4521-9   ISBN 978-1-4471-4522-6   (eBook)
DOI 10.1007/978-1-4471-4522-6
Springer London Heidelberg New York Dordrecht

Library of Congress Control Number: 2013947098

Printed on acid-free paper

Springer is part of Springer Science+Business Media (www.springer.com)

To Naomi, Freddie and Thea

About the Author

Jonathan Waxman is a Professor of Oncology at Imperial College London. He is a clinician who has helped develop new treatments for cancer, which are now part of standard practice. He is the founder and life president of Prostate Cancer UK, the first UK national organisation promoting research and patient support for this condition. He helped establish an All Party Parliamentary Group to improve cancer treatment and rationalise cancer research throughout the UK, and has developed and led several media campaigns to rationalise cancer treatments and change government health policy. '*MacLeod's Introduction to Medicine*', is his third fiction book and follows '*The Elephant in the Room*', and '*The Fifth Gospel*'.

www.jonathanwaxman.co.uk

Preface

This book is a collection of medical stories based on the epic career of MacLeod, its foolish hero. *MacLeod's Introduction to Medicine* is a chronicle of occasional humour, and the names of the characters have not been changed to protect the innocent. All the stories are based on reality and come from a time when the practice of medicine was not inundated with tales of bullying and scapegoating, where the lives of doctors, nurses and patients were not buried under targets and when the idiotic landslide of the internal market was on the other side of the mountain. It was only a little while ago that there was no overwhelming bureaucracy in the National Health Service and all who worked for the health of their charges did so with Joy, who was a lovely woman.

Jonathan Waxman
London, UK

Acknowledgements

My thanks as ever are to Naomi Heaton, and to Freddie and Thea Waxman for just about everything. I am also grateful to Harry Woolf, J G Ballard, Claire Walsh, Bob Brown, Cosmo Landesman, Maurice Slevin and Adrian Dannatt. I thank Teresa Dudley for this opportunity for publication and for her encouragement and adamantine support.

Contents

Contents

Chapter 1
The Grandest Surgeon

Sir Valentine Jenkinson-Smythe was a surgeon carved in the most traditional style. His early education at Harrow, where he was head boy, had been the prelude to First Class honours at Cambridge, where he was a rowing Blue. Cambridge was followed by a glorious medical school career at St Thomas's Hospital. Postgraduate success billowed and bulged, and he travelled on a Royal College of Surgeons' fellowship to Yale where his research on biliary obstruction was acclaimed on the international surgical stage. He specialised in gynaecology and his career blossomed. In his very early thirties he was appointed consultant gynaecologist to St Bartholomew's Hospital. He became a Freemason and his private practice flourished. He married well, to a gal of good family and even better fortune, and in time was appointed surgeon accoucheur to her Majesty, about whose private apartments he was most discreet.

With time, the svelte rowing Blue became a more substantial figure. Now, in his early sixties V J-S, as he was known to his colleagues, was portly and plethoric, his girth and complexion a product of fine dinners and fabulous wines, his stature at once reassuring and majestic. There was no one he reminded one of so much as George VI. In many ways, he was so like the king in manner, he lacked only an ermine robe for completion of the likeness.

J. Waxman, *MacLeod's Introduction to Medicine*,
DOI 10.1007/978-1-4471-4522-6_1,
© Springer-Verlag London 2014

V J-S was assiduous in the pursuit of his private practice, deigning only to descend to his NHS commitments at Barts in quiet moments when the grouse season was closed. In the evening, he could be found at his club, the Carlton, if anyone wanted to discuss medical school matters, but he retained his membership of the Reform for social events. He was a fierce clinical teacher who many thought had styled himself on the grandees of *Doctor in the House*. However, it is just as possible that Richard Gordon modelled Sir Lancelot Spratt on VJ-S. In a time when watch chains were unfashionable and when there were concerns about contagion in the wards, V J-S wore a chain across his double breasted pinstriped waistcoat, sported a carnation in his buttonhole and tramped through the hospital on his rounds wearing riding boots caked with mud.

If it had been possible to have a horse-drawn carriage take him to work, V J-S would have had one and it was to his chagrin that there was no stabling at Barts. V J-S made do with a Rolls-Royce instead of a carriage, and he took pleasure in driving the car himself. The Rolls was parked in the main square at Barts, where neither pigeon nor starling dared desecrate its polished carriage work.

'One would not have a chauffeur,' he boomed at a colleague, 'Not with a Rolls … but I would consider it, if I had a Bentley. Tell me, old chap, who of any breeding would have a Bentley?'

V J-S ran his firm on the most formal of lines. Medical students on his teaching team were seen to quake on his ward rounds, and hide behind each other when those fierce eyes looked to them for answers to his clinical questions. At his bidding, his juniors were often taken aside by their seniors and given advice on matters of tailoring or coiffeur. The advice was disregarded at peril of future career advancement. VJ-S thought that hair should be arranged as was appropriate to a young man of class and should not touch the ears nor fall below the collar, whilst a good tailored suit, three button, single vent, in a modest blue or grey was all that a man could ever need and represented a fine investment given that it could double for off-duty weekend wear.

At the end of each of his weekly ward rounds during the closed season, held in high pomp and with great ceremony, V J-S led his clinical team, senior registrars, registrars, housemen, Sister and medical students out of the wards, through the corridors and down the main stairs, towards the car park. As he walked, he continued the ward conversation, his words dragging his juniors behind him. And as he swept through the corridors, lesser mortals scattered and pressed themselves against the walls. Doors opened magically for him. V J-S's team hung on his opinions because their careers depended on his perception of them. His walk had a wake, a viscid stream of importance drifting from him and pushing all in his path out of his way.

V J-S's car rested majestically in a reserved parking spot in pride of place just by the main hospital doors. When he reached his car, in the shade of ancient plane trees, he engaged in caustic conversation with his team, berating them on matters of medical management. The doctors and nurses followed him in strict order of seniority, the senior registrar hanging on to V J-S's coat tails, the most junior of the housemen at the back of the parade. Getting into the Rolls and starting the engine, V J-S rolled down the window, continuing to chat. He put the car in gear and the Rolls moved forward.

The doctors and nurses walked beside the car keeping pace, helplessly caught in the net of his monologue, drawn in by his tirade. As his voice increased in volume, hectoring the registrar for some frightful misdemeanour, V J-S drove towards the exit, gently accelerating, head slightly inclined towards the most senior of his senior registrars, elbow pointing out of the window. The registrar stumbled in a pothole and fell, but the oblivious V J-S continued talking and, as he launched into a homily about the perils of pre-eclampsia, pressed down on the throttle. The car speeded up as did the attending juniors who accelerated as the Rolls gathered pace.

The line of medics, still ordered according to seniority, broke into a sharp trot, and then a smart run as the entrails of V J-S's story reached a climax. Senior registrars leading, junior doctors, medical students and nurses following, the doctors and nurses chased V J-S's car through the main square in a flurry of white coats and pinafores until the Rolls had driven out of the hospital and into Smithfield leaving doctors and nurses breathless in the wake of the car's exhaust.

V J-S was, of course, involved with all the hospital's great committees. There was no matter of any importance to the hospital's management that he didn't control. Most of the hospital's committee meetings were accompanied by liquid refreshments, and these were inevitably supplemented by more substantial provender. Refreshments were fundamental to the running of the committees for without sustenance very few of the hospital's great and good would have been persuaded to give up their time to serve on a committee. The selection of food and wine naturally required a further specialised committee and this, of course, V J-S chaired.

The Barts food and wine committee held meetings according to the time of year. There were evening meetings in the late autumn to select red wines, and lunchtime meetings in the spring to choose the white wines. The selection process entirely favoured Old World wine, for it was V J-S's view that nothing could be offered by the regions of viticulture beyond the French borders, and his view held sway over the views of lesser mortals.

There were twelve men on the wine committee. All had been at Barts for their entire working lives, all were Freemasons; there were no Jews and no black people on the committee – and there were certainly no women. Women were, however, allowed to serve the food, but not the drink from which the Barts' red wine list was to be chosen. The autumn wine committee dinner had been prepared in the kitchens that adjoined the Great Hall at Barts. The Great Hall is on the first floor of an eighteenth-century building designed by James Gibbs and is approached through an oak panelled hallway. Leaving their coats with the servants, the committee members strolled up the massive staircase of the building, leaning on the balustrade for support. The walls of the stairwell are highly decorated, painted opulently by Hogarth. Ignoring the beauty of their surroundings, as the committee members climbed the stairs to the Great Hall, they complained to each other en route about this and that insolent menial. Their destination was lit by chandeliers, there was stained glass in high windows and the ceiling was heavily plastered, its ornate pargeting a work of the highest skill.

In the centre of the hall was a dining table with two serving tables on each side. All three tables were clothed with gleaming white linen and dressed with silver, crystal and porcelain. Candles flickered in gilt candlesticks. On one of the side tables a legion of wine bottles was arranged in ordered lines. A tall thin man with a red nose stood nervously on guard, clasping his hands as he swayed from side to side, then backwards and forwards and finally from side to side again in a rhythmic yet random movement. This no doubt was Monsieur Rougenez, a vintner who had been brought in especially to service the Barts' committee's needs. From his shambling appearance, it seemed that although he may well have had a certain experience with wine, the degree of service that he might be able to provide to the Barts' consultants might be limited.

The wine committee was seated, with Valentine Jenkinson-Smythe enthroned at the head of the table. Conversation paused and grace was said. The clamour of conversation struck and V J-S tucked a voluminous napkin into his collar. The men seemed similar in demeanour and expression. They talked in a form of BBC English thought to have expired with their fathers, and taking up their implements they struck at their first course, pâté de foie gras. The pâté was served with a selection of three fine red wines, poured by the vintner. Each glass accompanying the hors d'oeuvres was filled to the brim, and the wine made a pretty display that contrasted delicately with the linen and cutlery.

M. Rougenez, presenting the wines to the club members, stuttered,

'These are Rhone wines, a perfect accompaniment to the foie ...

But he got no further, as V J-S, irritated by the man, interrupted in stentorian fashion,

'No need for any description, man, other than the name. The name of the wine. That'll be all, Sir.'

It was amazing to discover that a term of respect could be used in such a dismissive way, to which the good fellow gracefully replied,

'Of course, Sir Valentine. I suspect that you'll know far more than me about the wines.'

'Quite so.'

And the assembled worthies sat back in their chairs, tucked in to their meal and enjoyed the wines. Sorbets followed each course and these served to freshen the palates of the weary and rejuvenate the appetites of the gourmands. Conversation was hearty and at times rather crude. There was little focus on family but there was considerable interest in nursing staff and juniors. V J-S's neighbour was applauded for his story of a recent interview conducted for the appointment of a senior registrar in medicine.

'Confound the bloody college. Do you know what the devils had the impertinence to do? They insisted on the attachment of a college representative to the Appointments Committee. Clever chap, nice in his way, but an interfering do-gooder sort of so-and-so. You know the type?'

From the tenor of the general harrumphing and snorting that followed this question, it would appear that his friends did indeed know the type of person.

'In a way, I suppose that he was a decent sort of chap, but you know how they are? Anyway, the day for the interview comes along and we're in the board room. College fellow, and I do believe he may well have been a socialist, said that it's not really his place to get involved much in the detail of the interview but he did want to tell us that he was attending in order to see that due process had been followed by the Committee in its deliberations.

'Well, of course, the chairman thanked him for attending and noted his view. So on we went with the interview. There were six juniors to review. Excellent field. Five men, all with their FRCSs and all of them mind you, with doctorates, either MDs or MSs. The sixth, and in my view the most interesting, candidate was a woman, pretty thing about 5 foot 5, lovely, but no fellowship and no doctorate. So, of course, we gave her the job. We were unanimous. But then the College chappie piped up – he interrupted the chairman, damn cheek – and said, "Mr Chairman, I hope that you won't mind me commenting that the appointment hardly seems based on merit. The male candidates all have higher degrees and the woman does not."

'The Chairman turned to the college fellow and said – one has to admire his intellect –

'Dr MacLeod, thank you so much. An excellent point! But you must understand that we are old men. We need something attractive to get us through the day. We need something cheering on our ward rounds, old boy. It's in the interests of the hospital that we keep up morale, don't you know. With a lady registrar, operations will go smoothly because everyone will be doing their best so as to look good in front of the lady, and complication rates will fall. The appointment is to the advantage of the patients and staff. Thank you, though, Dr MacLeod. So kind of you to mention the matter.

'That sorted out the little squirt. You should have seen his face!'

As the applause and laughter subsided, the diners continued their meal, which was quite modest on this occasion – there were only seven courses. But the wines sampled were various and rich examples of the best of Bordeaux and Burgundy. Throughout the dinner, the waiters were at their posts behind the chairs of the wine club members, ever attentive to the needs of the great men. The tail-coated waiters stood to attention two steps behind the chairs of the gourmands, crisp white napkins folded neatly over the crooks of their right arms, splendid and virtually inanimate accompaniment to the cutlery and crockery.

There was little noise while the men ate; conversation was reserved for the spaces between the courses where proper attention could be paid to one's neighbour and respect given to position and place. In one such conversational lacuna, V J-S was minded of a surgeon under whom he'd had the pleasure to train and whose wit he admired greatly. V J-S turned to his colleagues and, undoing the bottom three buttons on his waistcoat, stretched out his legs and continued,

'Remember old Jolly Jerry, chaps? You know – Jerry, the general surgeon. Had five wives and seventeen children. Catholic, old Jerry, don't you know, and that I believe was the reason for the children but I don't think Catholicism could explain the five wives! Tremendous fellow, old Jerry, old school, you know the sort. Larger than life sort of chap he was. One thing you will remember about old Jerry was that he was a stickler for his private patients. He'd give them his best. Quite right, of course! They were paying for his services after all. Jerry would start his NHS operating list late. Reason was that he'd saved the NHS riffraff for the end of the day. Came to the hospital when he'd finished cutting up his private patients. Couldn't have the PPs running out of hours could he?

'Quite right! He absolutely had to give the private patients the best service. NHS are cut price after all! Cut price … surgeon … that's a joke, don't you know?'

A trickle of laughter rolled around the table, bounced onto the floor and tumbled down the stairs of the Great Hall.

'Anyway, back to the story. Jerry was operating. He was getting on with his NHS list. It was frightfully late. He'd got through the first three cases. There were another two cases to go. It must have been about 10pm and, of course, it was time for the nurses to change shift. They can't go on all night, women you know, not as tough as us men. Females! Goodness me! Wouldn't let them in to medical school if I had my way. Damn waste of public money. They're trained at vast expense, graduate, and then promptly get themselves pregnant! Lord, then you won't see them for dust. They're off and out of it, raising babies and then it's tea and sponge cake at the Women's Institute for the rest of their lives. Absurd! Madness! Simply bonkers! I wouldn't let a single female into medical school if I could have my way.

'Anyway I digress. Back to Jolly old Jerry and the theatre list. Night falls, old boy. Shift changes and the new nurses take over in theatre. Theatre Sister is an old-fashioned woman, don't you know, and the girlies have been taught how to behave properly …'

V J-S's audience had settled back in their chairs with brandy and port. An alcoholic mist had descended over the wine club and the men listened to him with a concentration that comes from twelve glasses of the best of Burgundy and Bordeaux and a well-fed stomach. The lights were dim in the Great Hall. The stoical waiters remained in attendance, and the man from the wine company could be seen in a far corner bent over a notebook mumbling as he totted up the evening's orders.

'The nurses hand over to each other and exchange information about the evening's list. You know how they do, checking this and that in case the blasted patient ends up going back to the wards with a retractor in his belly.'

V J-S's colleagues as one man, sensing a dénouement, sat forward in their chairs and turned to face the great man who continued,

'Scrub nurse having handed over said "Good night, Sir!" and scuttled awf, and the new scrub nurse introducing herself to Jerry as she had been taught, said,

'"Good evening, Sir, just to introduce myself. I'm Catherine, the relief nurse."

'And Jerry, quick as anything said, "Jolly good, hand or mouth?"'

The wine club members guffawed and V J-S, pleased with his friends' response to his anecdote, stood up and announced, 'I don't know about you chaps but I'm bushed. Time for home don't you know. Old lady's waiting. Better get back before dawn, whoever she is!'

And the great man stood up to go. At this the other club members stood too and all of them, much the worse for drink, staggered down the stairs, and wrestling with their coats emerged into the car park to find their chauffeurs. All except Sir Valentine who considered that there was absolutely no point in having a fine car and paying a ruffian to drive it for you.

V J-S fumbled in all of his pockets for his car keys, finding them eventually and reaching out clumsily for the lock opened the door of his Roller. He collapsed in the car seat, flexed his shoulders and tried to start the engine. After a little while, the engine fired up and he put the car in gear. The car launched backwards, bounced over the curb and stalled. V J-S started the car again. Waving good night to his friends, he sailed out into the night, the engine revving unnecessarily as he passed through the stone gateway that led out onto the main road that took him towards Smithfield.

It was midnight and the lamplight gleamed against an overcast sky. V J-S steered a course that held the nose of the Rolls over the white line in the middle of the road. The car lurched erratically as its driver tried to co-ordinate clutch and throttle. V J-S looked through the windscreen and the towers of Smithfield wobbled and swayed. He shook his head attempting concentration and the road ahead steadied itself. The entrance to Smithfield's meat market loomed and V J-S tacked back on a course that took him jerkily towards the narrow roadway that led through Smithfield to Farringdon and beyond.

The Rolls veered into the meat market. V J-S bumped over the curb as he lost his sight of the central white line. He lurched off the pavement and the car stalled again. Just as the engine coughed into life, a policeman loomed over the bonnet of the car and raised his right hand for V J-S to halt.

Through a bleary haze, V J-S noticed the policeman coming towards him and lowered the car window. The policeman stopped beside the Rolls, leaned forward and stared at Sir Valentine through the open window and recoiling at the coruscating shock of the driver's hyaena breath, said,

'Sir, your lights are switched off.'

Sir Valentine turned the car lights on.

'Very good! Well spotted, officer. Very kind. Thank you, my man.'

The policeman stroked his chin and reached for his notebook. Speaking with some care, he said, 'Sir, I have reason to believe that you have been drinking!'

Sir Valentine Jenkinson-Smythe, with back straight, half closed the car window against the cold of the night and the impertinence of the hoi polloi. He peered out into the darkness at the white face of the officer and frowned. V J-S pulled a handkerchief out of his pocket, blew his nose very loudly, and as he replaced his handkerchief in his sleeve, he replied, 'My dear fellow, I know your senior officer. Good night.'

The car window closed on the policeman and easing off the clutch, Sir Valentine and the Rolls-Royce coasted majestically out of Smithfield, making their stately way home, leaving the policeman scratching his head in their imperious wake.

Chapter 2
An Introduction to Medicine

It was fortunate for MacLeod that he had gone to the right sort of public school and providential that his father was a doctor. As a result of these two blessings, he was offered a place at medical school after a desultory interview that focused on his father's profession and MacLeod's inglorious school career.

At the end of a summer of love, a summer – mostly cold, wet and cloudy, a summer of love – mostly spurned, MacLeod took the tube from his North London home to Euston underground station. From there, he threaded his way through the tiny park that bordered Euston Station, sashaying around the piles of litter, the crushed beer cans and filthy cigarette butts that cluttered the leaf-strewn paths. He swerved past the leering, stumbling, rambling drunks, and after depositing coins in the hands of mumbling beggars, crossed the Euston Road.

As he made his way up Gower Street, MacLeod passed by the mucky entrance to Euston Square station and the begrimed doors and steamed-up windows of Lewis's medical bookshop on the corner of Gower Place. The traffic in Gower Street growled at the pedestrians on the zebra crossing and then roared south to the broken promises of Covent Garden. The wind swept a swirl of dust and leaves along Gower Street in haste to reach the City. As he strode along, MacLeod passed the classical stone portico of University College London, a portico redolent with promises of a grand education for all of its students. But MacLeod was oblivious to its

J. Waxman, *MacLeod's Introduction to Medicine*,
DOI 10.1007/978-1-4471-4522-6_2,
© Springer-Verlag London 2014

gleaming pillars and trumpeted promises because the carved Portland stone was obscured by the mists of anxiety that shrouded the morning of his first day at medical school.

Elsewhere in Gower Street, the autumn sun shone bright, and as MacLeod hurried along he looked at the faces of the young people walking with him wondering if they would be together on the same course. He faced a long haul through medical school and he knew that life as a medical student would be forged by hard work. He was aware that the first year and a half of his student life would be spent in pre-clinical sciences, learning anatomy and physiology, biochemistry and pharmacology, whilst the last three years of studentship would be spent as a clinical apprentice on the wards. But before the dawn of a life of study at UCL, MacLeod faced an introductory week – the exhausting razzle of an inebriated seven days and nights of freshers' parties.

MacLeod entered the medical school buildings en route to his first lecture which was to be held in the Biochemistry Lecture Theatre. Signposts pointed the way to the lecture theatre and he walked the corridors following the arrows that directed the new students to their 9.30 am introductory talk. In his hand, MacLeod grasped a rolled-up envelope that detailed the week's agenda. The envelope was damp with sweat. MacLeod's heart thumped, butterflies marched with hobnail boots through his intestines and his breath was quick.

MacLeod noticed that he was alone in the corridor; not a single new student followed his path and so he wondered if he had remembered the details of the day correctly. He stopped, opened the envelope and checked the introductory programme. He saw there in print what he already knew, which was that he was bang on schedule and in absolutely the right place. Putting the paper back in its envelope, he continued along the corridors to yet another signpost indicating that he was to take a left turn and then another telling him to turn right. And suddenly he had arrived; he had come to a dead end blocked by the Biochemistry Lecture Theatre's grand mahogany doors.

Double height and massively built, these doors were imposingly framed with bolection moulding and festooned with portentous, curlicued brass handles and elaborately engraved fingerplates. MacLeod hesitated at the doors, knowing that they would open onto a new phase of his life. During that pause, he briefly considered his life up to this point, reflecting that, given his background, the paths that he had followed had inevitably and so predictably led to this doorway to a new life. And then with a breath and a sigh, MacLeod considered his future, and wondered whether its corridors and doorways would have the inevitability and predictability of his route to medical school. Would he graduate, marry, have two kids, do his best for the people in his care, retire and die? Would his life be so entirely devoid of choice and so without freedom?

This pause for thought was but a moment's mote, and it was as if another MacLeod – an ageless MacLeod, independent of time and free of the tears of years, was observing him from high up, pressed tight to the peeling paint of the Biochemistry Department's ceiling. And was that lofty MacLeod looking down on that lowly MacLeod? And that other Ceiling-MacLeod; could he be seen staring at that Floor-MacLeod; and could he be observed to shake his head and smile knowingly at the smooth-faced youth below?

It felt to MacLeod as if this disembodied Ceiling-MacLeod was a keeper of his fortune, a surveyor of his road, the emperor that watched over his days, and as he, the Floor-MacLeod, aged, the man on the ceiling would not age, but would keep forever unlined and spry, the observer of his life, independent of the passing years.

MacLeod awoke from his daydream to find himself locked mid-stride, staring at the mahogany door's patina. From behind the doors there came a low buzz; the noise, the drone of the students beyond the doors waiting for him to enter their world. He hesitated, intimidated by the doors and the hubbub, intimidated by the thought of the significance of the change to his life that he was about to confront. MacLeod remained fixed at the door unable to push through the doorway, frightened by the prospect of his new life.

'Hello! Are you a new student, too?'

MacLeod turned to see a woman of his own age, short blonde hair parted on the right, a heart-faced, smiling woman dressed in an emerald green, two-piece silk suit, an outfit more appropriate for a debutante than a student.

'Yes!', he replied, in an urbane voice which he'd borrowed from someone he'd heard late night on the BBC's World Service.

'I think this is the place. Shall we go in?'

And with this, there was no option for MacLeod than to step bravely forward and proceed with the rest of his life. With manners dictated by the emerald girl's attire, he pushed the lecture theatre door open, and stood aside to let her in. As the heavy door opened they were engulfed by a tidal wave of laughter. Mocking shrieks buffeted them. Howling, hooting ridicule hissed from hordes of baying, hee-hawing students. Packed crowds of undergraduates stood up in the banked lecture theatre and roared their derision. Waving, shrieking, cawing, jumping up and down like deranged goblins, the students gesticulated at MacLeod and the emerald girl as they pushed into the lecture theatre. A Mexican wave of nightmare faces, name calling and laughter rippled through the theatre as MacLeod and Emerald stumbled in. They were caught in bright lights. Made rigid with fright they looked for a hiding place. In cacophonous rows of noise they sought a place of safety. They shuddered, and made catatonic with terror, they were catapulted into rigidity, framed by the doorway into the lecture theatre.

In that tumult, MacLeod wondered why the students were gawping and screeching at them? Was it their clothes, their hair? He looked for seats. They needed to get out of the spotlight fast. The students were hissing and howling, laughing and roaring, jumping up in their seats, screeching, caterwauling, pointing at them, banked-up rows of nightmare faces, shouting, gesticulating. They needed to get out of the limelight. Where could they find shelter? Where could they go to get away from the noise? The clamour was deeply personal, the embarrassment totally mortifying. They needed out of it. What an introduction to medicine.

MacLeod spotted two seats in one of the middle rows of the lecture theatre.

'Come on!', he said and grabbing Emerald's hand, he led her to the seats and sat down.

Still trembling after the ordeal, MacLeod held his face in his hands and bent forward in his seat, shaking with anxiety. After a few moments, he straightened up in his seat as the lecture theatre quietened. Silence was shovelled in to the auditorium by the sounds of a mocking hushing hissing from the students, a sardonic wind whooshing through the lecture theatre. Quiet was ushered into the room, and the sea of noise ebbed out into the Biochemistry Department corridors.

While he was recovering from the shock of the students' greeting, MacLeod turned to his partner but she seemed unphased by the brouhaha, and sat quite composed in her seat, absolutely relaxed and very cool. She pulled a silver powder compact from her handbag, flicked it open and looking at her face in its mirror, touched up her make-up. This was MacLeod's first contact with a teenager powder compact and he felt intimidated.

The students settled back, chatting quietly and as they did so MacLeod's equanimity gradually returned. But then suddenly the Lecture Theatre's door pushed open and a new student stepped into the room. Pimpled and tweed-jacketed, stooped and raw, the boy stumbled forward blinking into the dazzling lights of the lecture theatre. Instantly, the students jumped to their feet, shouting, cawing, pointing, screaming and the new student backed away trembling as the bristling broom of the old students' approbation swept him off his feet.

MacLeod felt no sympathy for the student, just relief that the ghastly tide of noise that had greeted his entry into medical school had not been personally directed, but the privilege of all who entered the university's portals. And what a privilege that was!

The day past more sedately after that first drooling-vampire-eats-the-newborn moment, filled by an introduction from the Dean and by various summaries of the curricula delivered by departmental heads. Over the course of freshers' week, MacLeod was introduced to the student clubs, began to make friends with beer and gained insights into life, the most important of which was that Guinness was unpleasant. In those seven days and nights, MacLeod made vital life-changing discoveries, such as the location of the student bar, where there was a table-football machine that was more popular than religion. In the beginning of that week, he also noticed that female medical students were an endangered species. And at the end of freshers' week, he came to the conclusion that most of the students in his year came from similar backgrounds to his; there seemed to be only one person from a working-class background.

Apart from a residual headache, the introductory week was over and it was time to begin coursework. The first lecture was entitled 'An introduction to anatomy'. The students sat waiting on tiered seats in the banked lecture theatre, looking down onto the lecturer's oak desk and the broad stretch of the blackboard beyond the oak desk. The clock hands swept to 9am. The minutes ticked by and it was 9.05, and then precisely on cue, exactly five minutes late, the doors to the theatre opened and the lecturer, Dr Zeki, shambled in, wearing blue jeans and an open-necked shirt, chest hair in bloom. He was short and balding, the morning's stubble thrusting out to greet the day. He walked with a big-bottom swagger, arms swaying, and stared at his audience, a gorilla's smile for all in the lecture theatre. He took up position behind the desk, planted his hands in his pockets, and leaning forward to his audience said,

'I'm going to tell you a joke,' Dr Zeki paused, smirked and nodded amiably at the first-year students.

Dr Zeki's audience looked at each other with disbelieving incredulity, and then sat back in their seats to listen.

'It's the first day of term at kindergarten.' Dr Zeki rested his finger tips on the desk, hesitated and glanced up at the ceiling lights.

'The children have a new teacher ... "Hello children!" says the new teacher. "My name is Miss Franny, and I do hope that you can manage to remember my name. For those of you who might have already forgotten, my name is Miss Franny and to help you remember my name, it's just Fanny, with an extra R. Miss Franny. So, repeat after me, children. Good morning, Miss Franny." And the good little children chorused, "Good morning, Miss Franny."

Dr Zeki relaxed into his joke. His hands retreated from the desk top and returned to his trouser pockets. He was enjoying himself. He liked the joke and he liked telling it. Dr Zeki scratched his pate. The medical students were bemused by their introduction to anatomy and wondered whether the rest of the lecture series would consist of jokes, and, if so, how exactly the exams would be marked. The joke continued.

'The day passed and at its end the children went home to their families. The next day came along and at 9 o'clock, the children, like the good little children that they were, assembled in Miss Franny's classroom ...'

Dr Zeki paused for dramatic effect and smiled at his audience. The hands came out of his pockets and MacLeod sensed that the joke's denouement was about to hit the lecture theatre fans, and hoped that the fan blades were strong enough to take it. The medical students listened attentively and Dr Zeki continued:

'Miss Franny smiled at the children sitting in front of her. Her smile was a sunshine smile, the sort that lights up a day. "Right, children!" she said. "I hope you're having a lovely day. You know how we start the day? Do any of you know how the day starts? You don't? Well children, we start with the register. I am going to take the register and I want you to say Yes if you are here and, of course, if you're not, you can keep quiet!"'

The medical students groaned and Dr Zeki's smile extended to the far corners of his face as he continued with his anecdote.

'"Great, that's wonderful children – no absentees. You're all here and that's a very good start to the day. Now children, let's see how good your memories are. Can any of you remember my name?"'

Dr Zeki paused and hesitated, and with that hesitation he appeared to concentrate and his smile extended even further to the tips of his ears. And with that pause, MacLeod knew that the lecturer was about to deliver the joke's punch line.

'The children bounced out of their seats, hands in the air, wanting to tell Miss Franny her name, and Miss Franny said, "Well done class, you all seem to know my name. Yes class, you may sit down. Sit down, please. May I have your answers, please? Yes, yes, I know you all know, but please could just one person answer at a time. Please sit down. Good. Now that you're sitting quietly, how about you, Sarah? Why don't you tell the class what my name is?"

'"Is it Mrs Smith, teacher?" No, Sarah. It is not Mrs Smith. Would anyone else like to tell me what my name is and look here's a big shiny red apple as a prize for anyone who can remember my name."'

There was complete silence in the lecture theatre. It was as if all the students were imaging themselves in Dr Zeki's Miss Franny's classroom. The medical students had become the kids trying to remember Miss Franny's name. The students strained forward attentively as Dr Zeki continued:

'"Sit down, everybody. Please sit down. You all get a turn. Ah, Johnny, little Johnny. Why don't you tell the class my name?"'

Dr Zeki folded his hands over his chest.

'Little Johnny stood up in class and smiled sweetly at his teacher. "I know Miss! I know!" "How clever of you to remember. What is it, Johnny?"

"Miss Crunt."'

Dr Zeki beamed at his audience, expecting applause, but there was no laughter. Silence greeted his punch line. The audience of blasé medical students was shocked by the profanity, shocked by the presence of the 'C' word, a word that was profoundly out of place and time.

Dr Zeki turned from his audience and stalked out of the lecture theatre. There was silence as the students gathered their things together. And then the silence was broken by hubbub, as the shocked students – amazed at the extraordinary 'lecture' – filed out of the room for a canteen coffee.

MacLeod found that Dr Zeki's lecture, although 'unusual' in the context of his education to date, was unremarkable in the context of the other lectures delivered by senior academics. There was little constraint and the lecturers' emphasis seemed to be on shocking the students rather than educating them. But as MacLeod mused, perhaps shock was an important component of his medical education.

The introductory course featured a talk from the Professor of Surgery, a talk planned, no doubt, to encourage the students contemplating the bleak hell of their pre-clinical subjects with the possibility that this dry desert would be followed by a paradise of enormous entertainment that would fill their clinical years. The first surgical lecture was delivered by Professor Charlie Clarke, who hurried into the lecture theatre. He was a very small man whose face was lined with nicotine's creases. He looked up at the medical students.

'Well, you bastards,' he growled, and continued, his accent, gruff Glaswegian.

'So, you think you want to be doctors? So, you think it's going to be just like the television programmes? Do you think it's going to be just like the telly? Well, let me give you an idea of the sort of stushie that will face you in Casualty!'

Professor Clarke paced the floor of the lecture theatre, his fingers curled around an imaginary cigarette.

'Imagine. It's 2 in the morning and there's a patient waiting for you to see him. Sister has called you to Casualty and you're there, you're the man on the spot. Now, imagine this. He's lying there in agony with abdominal pain. The abdomen, that's the medical term for the tummy, you bastards.

'So, what are you going to do about that? Well, I'll tell you what you do. You ask for an abdominal and pelvic X-ray. So, this is what happens. The patient's wheeled off to the X-ray Department and comes back having had his films taken, and what is it that you see at 2.30 in the morning? It's this, you bastards ...'

Professor Clarke's first slide flashed up on the screen behind him. The projected image was an X-ray.

'This is an X-ray of the man's abdomen and pelvis. Can anyone tell me what it shows?'

Professor Clarke's audience was quiet. No student offered a diagnosis.

MacLeod stared at the image. And saw there, centred low on the X-ray, the image of a beer mug, a ghost amongst the shadows, hiding within the shades of greys, whites and blacks.

Professor Clarke gesticulated impatiently at the students.

'One of you bastards, come on up. I want you to comment on the films. One of you step forward and point out what's wrong with the patient.'

No student volunteered. Professor Clarke pointed at a student sitting in the front row.

'You, boy! Come here!'

Boy was eating a bar of chocolate to Professor Clarke's evident irritation. Boy stumbled forward, and stood quivering in front of the screen, bar of chocolate melting in his hand.

'Well what do you think, you bastard?'

'I don't know, Sir.'

'Good. It's very good that you've admitted ignorance. That's an excellent start to your clinical career. Are you minded to admit any other deficiencies? Have you anything else that you wish to tell us?'

'No, Sir.'

'You may sit down, boy. Next, you, Sir. Yes, you with the stupid grin. Get up, come along, get up at once from that comfortable seat of yours. Get that big fat bottom of yours out of that chair. That's it. Get up,' and Professor Clarke waved him up from his seat in the back row, 'and let us have the benefit of your wisdom, you black-hearted bastard.'

There was no movement from the cowering medical students. Professor Clarke waved a billiard cue pointer at his audience, paced menacingly along the floor of the lecture theatre and gesticulated at his victim at the back of the lecture theatre, who flinched and then looked away from Professor Clarke.

'Yes, you, Sir. Don't look away, I am speaking to you. Yes, you, Sir. Please don't be shy. Step forward, young man, and give us the benefit of your opinion of this X-ray.'

The poor, intimidated student stepped timidly forward and, standing in the well of the lecture theatre, hands clasped behind his back, stared at the slide.

'I don't know what's wrong with the fellow, Sir, but the chap can't be all that well because he seems to have swallowed a beer mug, Sir.'

Professor Clarke had been intently watching the student as the man stared at the slide. He peered at him over the rim of his large rectangular tortoiseshell spectacles and slapped his thigh rhythmically with the billiard cue. Suddenly he leapt forward, waved the cue in the air and came to a halt two inches from the student who ducked as the cue swung over his head. The student shrank back, and cowered by the front row of seats bent double under the hissing arc of the billiard cue.

'Quite right, young man. You will go far. You got it in one go. Got it right, except for one thing. The patient didn't swallow the blasted mug. The wretched idiot shoved it up his bloody anus and couldn't get it out. And one other point ...

Professor Clarke turned to face his audience.

'In case any of you are wondering, it was a pint mug.'

The next slide flashed onto the screen. It was a penis, purple, engorged, bloody and horribly distorted.

The audience recoiled from the image of the mutilated member and gasped with horror.

'I'm not going to bother asking any of you what the object is on the screen because I know that you have led sheltered lives you Sassenach bastards.' Professor Clarke's audience of innocents relaxed.

'So, I'm going to tell you what it is. It's a blasted penis, you bastards, and it's been injured. And don't think that you have got away with it just because I've told you what it is that you are looking at. I can see you think that you can ride out this one but you cannot and you will not. I want you to tell me what is wrong with the offending item. Madam. Yes, you Madam. Step forward. Yes, now come along. Come to the front. That's it. Now, step up to the screen. Don't be shy.'

Professor Clarke waved his cue at Emerald, who it turned out had a proper name – Leticia Clements – and that proper name was about to be revealed.

'What is your name?'

'Clements, Sir.'

'Ah. A good start to the course. You know your name and I trust you can also manage to spell your name. If you can do so, you will go far, Madam. So, Madam. Can you tell me what is wrong with this penis?'

Professor Clarke bashed the screen with his billiard cue.

Leticia stepped closer to the screen and stared at the penis.

'Can't tell, Sir, but it does look awfully sick.'

'You are right, Madam. And you need go no further. I will enlighten you. Sit down. Yes. You can sit down, Madam. You may now go back to your seat. Yes, Madam, go back to your seat now, there's a good boy, Madam.'

Professor Clarke spun on his heels and thrashed down through the air with the billiard cue. He whacked the desk and then half turned to the screen and smacked the billiard cue on to the projected penis which buckled under the blow.

'This, you bastards, is another Casualty Friday night special. What you see before you is a vacuum cleaner injury. You know why this idiot of a patient ended up in Casualty? The stupid bastard told us that he was doing a bit of housework, and slipped onto his Hoover. There is no way that he could possibly have done himself that sort of amount of damage by simply slipping. The bastard was getting himself sucked off by the blasted vacuum cleaner!'

There was a profound intake of air in the lecture theatre, the medical students horrified by the crudity and unexpectedness of the professor's language.

'Yes,' mumbled Professor Clarke, in an unpleasant growl, 'and here's the thing. The fool sat at home nursing the damage and didn't come right in and get himself looked at. By the time that he got to Casualty, gangrene had set in and we had to cut it off, the stupid bastard. And let that be a lesson to you all. Never, never, never, under any circumstances, agree to do housework on a Friday night!'

Professor Clarke slapped the billiard cue down on the desk, and as the cue rolled off and clattered onto the floor, he strode out of the lecture theatre, muttering ...

'Black-hearted Sassenach bastard.'

... and leaving his audience wondering who exactly the bastard was.

MacLeod's physiology classes were led by a starry group of scientists. There were Nobel laureates in the university, Professors Huxley and Katz, and other eminent scientists whose names were attached to theories that were of world renown. Hugh Davson was one of the UCL scientists whose work had achieved international recognition. His studies had led to the eponymous Davson-Danielli theory of membrane structure, a theory that could be spotted on the tip of everyone's tongue everywhere you went in the Western world. MacLeod was in awe of these scientists; they were superstars in his view, superstars who were mostly quiet in their ways, unlike the footballers and hairdressers wrestling for the limelight.

MacLeod sat in the front row for Dr Davson's first lecture. He was curious to know how he looked and talked. MacLeod wanted to focus on this scientific éminence grise, and was prepared to watch him in action for hours and hours. As the second hand on the lecture theatre clock tiptoed into position, Professor Davson marched into the lecture theatre. His demeanour was immaculate: straight back, clipped moustache, short hair. He was beautifully dressed, be-suited, with a gleaming white handkerchief folded neatly into his top pocket. But amidst all that was conventional, there shone a certain twinkle. He greeted the students with a crisp 'Good morning', then he turned to the board to write a few notes.

'These points summarise my lecture. You won't need anything else. Do copy them if you wish.'

There was quiet in the lecture theatre as the students copied from the board. In a few brief words that filled grammatically correct sentences of admirable concision, Professor Davson explained how cell membranes were formed. After only a few minutes, MacLeod was left with an amazingly clear understanding of the structure of the cell membrane. The explanation was so good that it seemed like the most extraordinary enlightenment. There was silence in the lecture theatre as Professor Davson crooked his left arm and with a twist of his hand exposed a gold watch.

'Ah, it is 12.15.'

The lecture had been scheduled from 12 to 1 pm.

'That's quite enough for the day. Lunchtime, I think. Good day to you.'

There was an amazed, jaw dropping, vacuous silence from the students as Professor Davson walked out of the lecture theatre, and as he left MacLeod thought,

'What a sensible fellow. No student absorbs much after the first fifteen minutes of a lecture. The rest of the lecturer's time is usually wasted. He'd said what was needed to be said! And he's right – it's lunchtime. What a genius.'

The students left the theatre shaking their heads, many thinking they'd been swindled because Professor Davson's talk had been so brief, but MacLeod knew otherwise.

Chapter 3
The Pleasures
of Undergraduate Research

In their first years of medical school, students are taught the basic science that underpins their clinical studies: anatomy and physiology, biochemistry and pharmacology – and so MacLeod spent the flower of his youth sitting around a stinking corpse and loitering in laboratories. In the dissection room, groups of medical students clustered around twenty yellowed bodies laid out on steel tables. There, under neon light in a gloomy basement, the students breathed in foul formaldehyde-tainted air and mapped out brown and yellow planes of fascia and aponeuroses, and stringy cords of blood vessels and nerves. Muscle groups and bones were put on display like so many proud leeks and onions at a WI harvest festival.

MacLeod seemed to live in laboratories, where scalpel blades were at play picking out the arterial systems of rats, and electrodes tormented the nervous system of frogs pinned out on teak worktops. He learned about blood – its red cells and its white cells, platelets and plasma staring at him from a pink droplet on the glassy surface of a microscope slide. There were biochemical pathways to discover; neural networks and physiological cascades, maps of brains and arteries, psychologies and histories, interactions and sensitivities, inflammation and malignancy. Neurotransmitters, drug interactions, temperature regulation, appetite and oxygen sensors, autonomic regulation and pain perception, reflexes and viruses, cholinergic and adrenergic receptors, mitochondria

J. Waxman, *MacLeod's Introduction to Medicine*,
DOI 10.1007/978-1-4471-4522-6_3,
© Springer-Verlag London 2014

and nuclei, antibiotics and immunity, electrodes and pipettes, kinases and the sodium pump.

And MacLeod found that medicine was a great education, a way to the world, an explanation of how things worked. Medicine was the road to science, the route map to discovery; it was an exploration of the nature of man, an elucidation of the mechanics of mankind. In the early days of his course, MacLeod was in love with his studies, the minutes and hours, days, weeks and months spent with books as his best friends, learned journals as his soul mates, reference works as his dearest companions.

MacLeod's studies were a magnet, a force of attraction that clasped the keen medical student to its heart and embraced him, clothed him in the beauty of knowledge; beauty that amazed and dazzled him. But all forces have their opposites, dark has light, positive has its negative and for that force whose South Pole was 'knowledge', MacLeod's North Pole was 'play'. And in the student bar and the discos, in the parties and clubs, MacLeod discovered … girls.

MacLeod found that he spent less and less time at work as the months and the terms of his course shunted by. And so it came to pass in his second year at Medical School that instead of dark hours in dusty libraries bent over his books, MacLeod spent his time partying. The balance of his life shifted and work became a trivial nuisance, moments spent cramming just enough information to get by.

And yet, during this second year of university, in the dark lacunae of time unoccupied by his social life, MacLeod found himself once more captivated by his course. He turned again to study, enjoyed again the company of books. He became interested in his medical training; he found peace in his books and fascination in the science and art of medicine. This change surprised both his fellow students and his teachers. All were astonished to observe that he had become as assiduous in the pursuit of learning as he had been in his pursuit of girls. There were differences, of course, between girls and books and this MacLeod had learned quite early on in his medical school career. For example, he found that books made no effort to escape from his clutches whereas girls made no effort to enter his clutches. There were other differences, too; MacLeod found satisfaction in his life with books which is more than could be said that he found in his life with women.

The months turned and a summer of love came into view, a summer without sun because all light was overshadowed by the black cloud of exams. And not just any exams; it was the mother of all exams, Second MB, the watershed where pre-clinical studies ended and clinical life began. Second MB was a serious exam; there was not a trace of flippery nor flimflam to the examination. Failure meant that students could not progress to hospital life. A fearsome amount of work, but no intelligence whatsoever, was required to pass Second MB. Students had to cram as much information as possible into their brains, with the hope that the surfeit of information would spill out and onto the terrifyingly blank pages of the exam question papers. In the weeks leading up to the exams, the library, a previously undiscovered destination for the majority of medical students, became crammed with assiduous youths anxiously cramming for their Second MB.

MacLeod loved the medical school library, a parade of panelling, where crowds of ancient books gossiped in oak galleries. There, in the heights, the tomes gathered and crumbled, living lives of peace that were generally undisturbed by students. On shelves of dust, leather-bound knowledge sat ready and waiting, promiscuous, available, free to be had by one and all, but never really troubled for their favours.

The medical students sat at lines of desks wearing out their elbows, bowed heads peeping over mounds of screwed-up paper. From the heights of the library, alabaster and marble busts of great physicians and surgeons – Victorians, Georgians, Edwardians, admired for their baldness, competing in their exuberant facial hair – looked down on the students at their desks. The statues' facial features struggled through antique forests of glorious moustaches, peered through tumbling copses of eyebrows, poked through beards and side whiskers. Pebble eyes peeped down at the new generations of students.

In the silence of the library, was it possible to hear the muttered whispers of the great stone men, rippling down from the heights of the bookshelves? In the fractured silence, did sharp criticism echo, noisy comment on the idle lives of the students below?

In the ghostly galleries of the library, the librarians shuffled, pushing trolleys stacked with returned books, and on mezzanine shelves placed books and stacked periodicals, filling galleries of information, organising a world of knowledge on death and disease. Bent over their laden trolleys, pushing their books before them, they were like dinner ladies, although their load was a nourishing concoction of well-seasoned knowledge rather than skinny custard and stinking stews!

Exam time came duly rolling by, and an anxious MacLeod shuffled into the windy exam hall, and took his place amongst the rows of nervous medical students. An invigilator with a handlebar moustache paraded before the students.

'Right!' he boomed as he strode backwards and forwards, pacing the exam hall.

'Right, you horrible bunch of doomed fools. Now listen up and listen up good. You will know that there is an absolute requirement for all students to bring textbooks into the examination hall.' The invigilator threw a piece of chalk at a light fixture, pirouetted on his toes and continued,

'And furthermore, you have already been informed by the authorities of the need to communicate between friends during exams, the fixed requirement not to stick to time, and the additional points to be gained from copying colleagues' answers.'

The invigilator stroked his moustache and fumbled in his pockets, and then the bell to start the first of the exams struck and rang out through the hall.

In a flush of terror and panic that filled his days, MacLeod's examination fortnight rolled by. The papers were marked and the day finally arrived when the results were due. On that sunny June morning, MacLeod took the tube train to college to line up with his peers around a notice board in the student common room. A list of the successful exam candidates was posted on this gloomy cork board.

Medical students crowded around, pushing against each other in their anxiety to find their numbers. The presence of his number on the board indicated that the candidate had passed his Second MB. The absence of a number denoted failure. The students searched for their numbers, breath held, attention fixed on three sheets of peeling A4 pinned to the centre of the board, three white sheets surrounded by garish posters advertising end of term student balls and rooms to let. The students scanned the printed columns of numbers. These were in order, starting at the top of the page with '1' and finishing at the bottom with '240'. Students searched the list, looking for their candidate number, and then withdrew from the tumult with a sigh or a cheer. And then each student returned to check the list to make sure that their eyesight hadn't been deceived by nightmares and dreams.

MacLeod's number was on the list. He staggered back and collapsed in a chair, unbelievably relieved and then, like all the other students, pushed back into the melee to check that he had really seen his number on the board. He checked his exam number on his candidate slip, looked up again at the list and decided that it was time for a trip to the bar. Once there, he found lines of medical students clamouring for beer – solace for failure and lubrication for success. It was 9.30 am and everyone in his year, without exception, needed a drink.

As MacLeod staggered home, tipsy to the extent that he had travelled several stops in the wrong direction on the Northern Line before noticing that he was heading south and not north towards home, he was confronted with the realisation that he faced a whole summer with nothing planned. He had spent so much time studying that he had failed to organise a holiday or employment to fund that holiday.

'So,' he wondered, 'what shall I do?'

Now, although MacLeod had spent a considerable part of his student life having fun, he'd also spent time working hard, enjoying his studies almost as much as his social life. He'd been fascinated by biochemistry and, in particular, by the emerging world of molecular biology. For MacLeod, there was entrancement in ribosomes and excitement in mitochondria. The way that genes worked and their potential importance in the control of disease seemed to him to be the way of the future. It had been stimulating for MacLeod to consider how genetic mutation could cause cancer in children, although that revelation wasn't going to please those affected. And he was certain that the way ahead for medicine lay in a greater understanding of how genes worked.

These were early days in the discovery process of molecular biology and insights into the mechanisms that lead to the development of disease were still to be revealed. There seemed to be nothing more important to him than trying to understand how cancer evolved, and he was certain that his career in medicine would end in specialisation in cancer research.

In his student life, MacLeod had become friendly with Dave Williams, his biochemistry tutor. They got on and it seemed to MacLeod that his tutor observed the high jinks of student life with wistful amusement. Dave was about 40 years old. He had straight sandy brown hair parted at the side, John Lennon-style glasses, a goatee beard and a twinkly smile that owed a lot to his glasses catching reflected light. Dave always wore a tatty, leather-patched tweed jacket with corduroys and brothel creepers. MacLeod wouldn't have been surprised if Dave wore tweed to bed as he'd never seen him without his jacket. Dave Williams was fun; he was sardonic and very clever. His office was on the ground floor of the Biochemistry Block, and MacLeod went to see him soon after the exam results.

'Hey Dave. I'd love to work for you. Can you give me something to do over the summer holidays, please? I want a project; you know, research. And what I really want to do – I'm being serious about this – is to cure cancer. You're a clever fellow, Dave, but I don't think that you've been applying yourself enough. With you and me on side, working together, getting serious, I think that we've a good chance of making it big. What I think is possible, and I've thought about this a lot, Dave, so don't get me wrong here – don't think I'm just a lightweight, because I really have given the subject some attention – what I think is possible – is to find the cause of cancer in one biochemical experiment. Dave, so tell me, have you got anything that would fit the bill?'

Dave Williams nodded, tugged at his beard and, looking up from a desk heaped high with books and covered with papers, grinned at MacLeod. The sun bounced off his spectacles, momentarily blinding him.

'Sure. I have just the project for you. It'll take you about six weeks and we'll pay you a paltry sum, my boy, but it'll keep you in beer and fund the occasional trip to the cinema. What do you think?'

MacLeod didn't need to think.

'Great. Thank you, Dave!'

MacLeod was thrilled at the thought that he could work with his favourite academic and find out something that existed beyond the textbooks.

Dave leaned forward and clicked into serious mode. He was about to lecture MacLeod and MacLeod sensed that he wasn't going to stop until he had drawn the lecture to its conclusion.

'This is what I want you to do, MacLeod. It starts with this, my boy. We know that there are differences in the hormonal profiles of women with breast cancer that antedate the development of their cancers. Prospective studies on closed populations of women in the Channel Islands have shown that the differences in female hormones predicate for the development of breast cancer.'

MacLeod started to slump in his seat, but Dave Williams was not going to stop for anything. His attention was on his subject, not MacLeod, and he stood up, waved his arms in excitement and warmed to his subject.

'We can use a formula based on the ratio of the different female sex hormones in urine to identify those women at risk of breast cancer. Now MacLeod, you will know from your Second MB that the precise balance of sex steroids can cause changes in the ratio of free to bound ribosomes, which you'll remember from your Second MB, is the machinery for synthesising messenger RNA, and that a decrease in bound RNA is associated with cancers.'

Dave paused and looked at MacLeod, wondering if he was getting his drift. MacLeod smiled engagingly and so Dave, encouraged by MacLeod's pretence at interest, continued:

'What I'd like you to do is collect breast tumours from the operating theatre. You'll have to stand in theatre whilst the surgeons are operating because if you don't, then they'll forget that we want their specimens – they've memories like walruses. Now as soon as they are removed, put the tumours in dry ice so that the metabolic processes are put on hold.

'Now, this is the important bit, MacLeod, it's when the science starts. Focus, MacLeod! Focus! I'd like you to bring the tumours back to the lab and go on to assay free and bound ribosomes. We will measure the levels of sex hormones in the women with cancer and see if there is any correlation between hormone levels and the ratio of free to bound ribosomes.'

MacLeod nodded at the beaming academic, but he had absolutely no idea what the man was talking about.

'We have the system set up. John Wiley, the breast surgeon, wants to help by providing us with the breast tumours. What do you think? Would you like to help on the project?'

Of course, MacLeod would like to help with the project. In his dreams he wanted to be a cancer researcher – he felt that this was going to be his life's work. And as he left Dave William's office, he found himself whistling along the basement corridors and out into the Gower Street sunlight.

In theatre the following week, MacLeod, in surgical scrubs, waited patiently behind Mr Wiley, who leaned over the anaesthetised towel-draped body of a woman with breast cancer. Mr Wiley glanced back at MacLeod. A surgical registrar held a trembling retractor at the ready, the anaesthetist lolled, legs crossed, reading a newspaper, and the nursing Sister watched anxiously over the proceedings, a roll of gleaming surgical instruments in front of her on a green surgical drape, ready for the surgeon's demands.

Mr Wiley commented for his trainee's behalf on his surgical technique in an exaggerated Scottish burr as he cut through skin to the layer of yellow fat below.

'There – no blood at all. That's how you do it. Oh goodness – there's a bleeder!'

And with a fizz, Mr Wiley poked at the tiny subcuticular blood vessel spouting bright blood and cauterised the arteriole. The bleeding immediately stopped and, as the fountain of bright blood collapsed, the smell of burnt flesh wafted through the operating theatre. MacLeod leaned forward concentrating on the operation, ready to take the tumour from Mr Wiley as soon as it was removed from the patient. The patient's chest heaved up and then down, puffed by the mechanical tide of the respirator. The anaesthetist turned to more important things, ignoring the patient and flicking through the pages of *The Times*, checked his share prices. He reached down to the anaesthetics' trolley, grabbed a pencil, then wetted the point on the tip of his tongue and started on the crossword.

'Pull back on that retractor, man!' hooted Mr Wiley.

The registrar opposite Mr Wiley started, and then did as ordered.

Mr Wiley looked up from the scene of operation and stared at an X-ray box with a mammogram clipped to it, which gave the surgeon a view of the tumour. There, outlined on a black and white A4 image of the patient's breast in profile, a clump of chunky white specks was starkly highlighted against a grey-streaked background of normal breast tissue. The clump of specks defined the location of the cancer. The surgeon looked up at the mammogram and then down at the woman's breast assessing where to place his incision, matching X-ray changes with breast topography. His eyebrows drew together as he concentrated, cutting through normal breast tissue around the mass of tumour. MacLeod clutched at the white polystyrene container that held the carbon dioxide ice that was to be the home for the tumour on its journey to the labs.

'There it is!' Mr Wiley exclaimed, as he pulled gently up at the breast mass. 'It's out.'

And Mr Wiley pulled the tumour from the breast, as though it were a bloody rabbit removed from the magician's hat. The surgical registrar tidied the wound, sewing the edges of tissues together while Mr Wiley placed the mass of tumour in a kidney dish. Then the surgeon cut into the lump of flesh with his scalpel neatly bisecting it.

'There,' he said, turning to MacLeod. 'Here's the bastard! Can you see how different it is from normal tissue?'

MacLeod, hovering over the metal kidney dish stared at the specimen as Mr Wiley poked at it with his scalpel.

'Look, MacLeod. Can you see that the cancer is paler than the normal surrounding fat?'

MacLeod could see that the tumour was indeed whiter in colour than the yellow fatty tissue that surrounded it.

'And can you see that, as I cut into it, it's much harder than the normal tissue around it?'

MacLeod stared into the kidney dish and could easily see how different the tumour was from the surrounding breast tissue. The cancer looked like a pear in shape, colour and consistency, and although it appeared well demarcated from the surrounding breast, he could see that strands of tumour branched off from the main mass of the cancer and crept into adjacent breast tissue. The 'pear', red flecked and oozing blood, lay in the kidney dish like an alien thing that had lost its spaceship.

Picking up a pair of forceps, Mr Wiley grasped half of the tumour and laid it on the ice in MacLeod's polystyrene box.

'There you are, MacLeod. Off you go to the labs and do your stuff.'

MacLeod did as he was bid and scurried out of the operating theatre suite. Braving the winds of Gower Street, he crossed the road to the Biochemistry Department. In the labs, he stared at the tumour at rest in a glass dish on a bed of dry ice, and considered with wonder how such a small mass of tissue could cause death and destruction. He cut the cancer into small pieces with a scalpel and tweezers. Then, using a sonic probe, he macerated the tumour, smashing it up into tiny pieces.

Next, MacLeod had to separate out the cellular components of the tumour using a method that involved spinning the tumour fragments in an ultracentrifuge. This method exploited the fact that each cellular component has a specific density and so can be precipitated at different spin speeds. By this means, MacLeod would be able to get at the particular cellular elements that he needed for the next stage of his experiment. MacLeod divided the tumour fragments into equivalent portions and then loaded the portions into glass centrifuge tubes. He added solvents to the tubes and, carefully weighing them on scales, made sure that they were exactly the same weight as each other so that they would spin without destroying the ultracentrifuge. If the tubes were just a jot out of balance, this difference in weight would be exaggerated at high speeds and destroy the ultracentrifuge's rotor.

The ultracentrifuge was a gleaming green beast that lurked in the basement of the Biochemistry Department. It loomed gloomily in its basement corner sulking like an ominous washing machine that was up to no good. MacLeod screwed down the lid of the centrifuge and set it to spin – it was capable of speeds up to 80,000 rpm. The machine throbbed and hummed as its rotor accelerated to higher and higher speeds, and then finally settled to an even rumble.

MacLeod left the centrifuge to do its duty, and went for a coffee. Coffee was his friend, warm and sweet. He sat in the common room reading *The Times*. He turned first to the Obituaries section, the 'Register'. He enjoyed reading these stories of the dead. Those who had striven and loved and done this and that, and begat and sometimes hadn't even married. But what in the end was the product of their days? MacLeod really had no idea at all.

The centrifuge was set to spin for forty-five minutes. MacLeod had a pocket alarm in his lab coat set to remind him when the machine was due to stop. The little timer whirred and clicked through the minutes. Time was up and the alarm rang. MacLeod washed his mug in the grimy sink and returned to the centrifuge room through the basement corridors. As he entered the room, the rotor was gently slowing, whistling down through the octaves as it came juddering to a halt. The centrifuge stopped with a shudder, and the room was suffused with silence broken by a click as the machine's safety release switched off.

MacLeod opened the centrifuge lid, unscrewed the cover and pulled his tubes from the rotor head. Then he returned to the lab to carry out the final stage of his experiment where he re-suspended the pellet at the bottom of the centrifuge tubes and assayed smooth and rough endoplasmic reticulum. The complexities of the assay results, spewed out though lines of equipment, dials and needles, through monitors, connected by wires and bulldog clip contacts, were recorded on a roll of temperature-sensitive graph paper, inscribed by the touch of a heated needle. This traced a line on the paper and the position of the black line on the graph paper enabled a calculation to be made of the relative amounts of smooth and rough endoplasmic reticulum.

The experiment trundled to a close and MacLeod tore off the yard of graph paper on which his results were recorded and wrote the date and tumour sample numbers on the paper. He waited for the ink to dry and then folded away the paper into a nice blue filing box that he'd bought specially for his project.

In the days that followed, MacLeod spent hours in the medical records department looking up patient details in their hospital notes. And he recorded lists of the clinical characteristics of his patients, hoping to correlate his results with details of his patients' ages and hormone levels, and information about the microscopic features of their tumours. He knew that at the end of his summer project he would have to go through his observations with Dave Williams. MacLeod enjoyed the rhythm of his work, the specimen collections in theatre, the banter with the surgeon and the nurses, the assays, but most of all he loved his coffee breaks.

At the end of his summer project, MacLeod reviewed his findings with his supervisor. Dave Williams sat behind his desk and MacLeod sat facing him. Since MacLeod's initial request for work, the pile of papers and books on Dr Williams' desk had increased in height such that he could barely be glimpsed behind tottering volcanoes of paper. The office walls were clothed with heavily laden bookshelves that creaked and swayed. Through the mass of papers, his back against a wall of books that tottered alarmingly over him, Dave Williams appeared to be boxed into a paper cave of his own making, a cave lined with the industry of his life. The room was gloomy. August had mired the office windows with dust and dirt. The basement windows were opened to the Gower Street breeze and clatter of traffic.

'Well, MacLeod, have you had a good summer? I guess these are your results that you've brought me?'

Dave Williams stood up and reached over the hillocks on his desk for the filing boxes that MacLeod had brought to show him.

'Yes, Dr Williams.'

'Jolly good.'

Dave Williams swept lank hair from his forehead and opened one of MacLeod's boxes. His face crumpled with concentration as he pulled out the reams of notes that MacLeod had made on the characteristics of the patients and their tumours. Clasping both filing boxes to his tweedy chest, he sat down abruptly on the edge of his desk and a pile of his papers tumbled on to the floor, pushed to one side by his bottom. But Dr Williams, oblivious of the landslide, focused on MacLeod's documents and shuffled through the sheets of paper.

'Good, that's very good. You've captured all of the information that we'll need to make an analysis.'

Dr Williams stuffed the papers back into the first filing box and looking around for a space on his desk for it, and finding there was none, flung the box at MacLeod.

'Well caught, that man!'

Dr Williams opened the second filing box and unrolled tightly wound sheets of recording paper. He inspected the pen recording traces with interest, his eyes squinting as he took in the complexities of the spidery line that trickled along the graph paper. He followed the line with his Gauloises-stained index finger and then scratched his chin. He turned the paper upside down and followed the course of the heat tracing again, trying to establish its significance. His interest turned to puzzlement. Dr Williams put down the heat trace and extracted another roll of paper from the filing box.

'Interesting ... interesting.'

Dr Williams snapped both boxes shut, clutched them to his chest, paced the small office, and after walking around his desk, sat down with a great sigh that was echoed by air exhaled by his chair cushions. He swept aside various piles of papers on his desk, placed the filing boxes in the clearing and unravelled another pen recording.

'Very interesting, very interesting indeed.'

And his nicotine-stained fingertip again prodded at the pen recording following the heat trace as it wandered across the close lined squares of the scroll.

MacLeod couldn't understand what his supervisor was doing. Certainly, Dr Williams seemed interested in his results, but he hadn't made any specific comment about the meaning of his observations. He had said that the results were interesting, but something wasn't right. MacLeod felt anxious. Dr Williams pondered over the recordings, darting from one to another without specific comment, his finger following the lines, his head bent over the recording paper. Tension levels rose in Dr Williams' office and MacLeod shifted uncomfortably in his seat.

'What's he up to?' MacLeod puzzled.

Then suddenly a smile creased Dr Williams' face. He looked up from MacLeod's recordings. His grin spread and, behind those John Lennon spectacles, his eyes glimmered with amusement.

MacLeod was even more puzzled, and thought to himself,

'What's he up to? What's going on? What on Earth is so funny about my results? I've worked hard for them. What's the matter with the bastard? Why is he grinning?'

'Now look here, MacLeod. You do know what you've done, don't you?'

MacLeod had no idea what he'd done. No idea at all. He shook his head and waited to be told.

'MacLeod!' Dr Williams waved a handful of pen recording paper at him and roared with laughter. 'My dear chap, you know what you've done?'

MacLeod hadn't a clue.

'You've been picking up Radio 1 on the pen recorder. That's what this is. Radio 1.'

Dr Williams collapsed back in his chair roaring with laughter and MacLeod hung his head with disbelief.

'What a waste of a summer!'

'Not at all. Don't worry MacLeod, all will be well. You've worked hard. These results are more a commentary on my supervision than your lack of scientific skill. I should never have left you alone with all those test tubes. But we'll sort it out. You may not get a scientific paper out of the work but I will put you in for a medical school prize. How do you fancy the Thomas Lewis Prize for medical research? You deserve it!'

Dr Williams got up from his desk, stuffed MacLeod's papers in an overflowing rubbish bin and clapped his student on the back.

'Fabulous. Just excellent, lad. Great stuff!'

And with that slap on the back, MacLeod's misery dispersed. He realised that he had learned a precious lesson. In that moment, he understood the value and nature of scientific research. He knew that the holiday project had been a wonderful experience that had informed him forever about the essence of scientific endeavour. It was clear to MacLeod that if ever he turned to research again he would check always check his leads first.

But, as you might imagine, that wasn't quite the end of MacLeod's life in medical research. However, it was a good start to the rest of the summer spent in the Greek Islands and a return to clinical studies that ended with many other glorious prizes and scholarships that decorated his curriculum vitae and added several inches to his manhood. These prizes, scholarships and particularly the extension to his manhood ensured that, at qualification, MacLeod's fate would be sealed. He would be doomed to suffer the trials and tribulations of a career in academic medicine.

Chapter 4
In Foreign Parts

'Would you like a lift home, MacLeod?'

The offer was from MacLeod's physiology tutor, Professor Bernard Katz. MacLeod was eighteen years old and Professor Katz was around sixty, but with his wattles and wrinkles, his thick spectacles and old-fashioned suit, he seemed considerably older than his years. In contrast, MacLeod, with his spots and baby face seemed considerably younger than eighteen. However, MacLeod and Katz had a few things in common. For example, MacLeod lived at home with his parents and Professor Katz also still lived at home, though obviously not in the same home as MacLeod nor with his parents! Professor Katz's home was just around the corner from his student's home. Knowing this, the professor had kindly offered MacLeod a lift after a tutorial group at the end of a fine summer's day.

Professor Katz was a biophysicist who had contributed hugely to the science of cellular communication. He had made observations about the nature of the impulse that travels between nerve and muscle cells. In 1970, he would be awarded a Nobel Prize in recognition of his extraordinary work. Life had hardly been easy for Bernard Katz. He had escaped from Leipzig in 1935 and avoided being massacred by the Nazis – one of the few Jews who had escaped the wartime genocide in central Europe. Professor Katz was part of that amazing nucleus of central European Jews who gave so much to the world. He had survived; so many had died – and

J. Waxman, *MacLeod's Introduction to Medicine*,
DOI 10.1007/978-1-4471-4522-6_4,
© Springer-Verlag London 2014

MacLeod wondered what the world would have been like, if not for the decimation reaped by the Holocaust.

Although the tutorial had ended for the majority of the tutorial group, its themes continued as MacLeod and Professor Katz strolled through the college's corridors. As they walked, the professor talked and MacLeod listened, enjoying the densely *mittel*-European flavours of Professor Katz's accent, as the great man enthused over his subject.

MacLeod and Professor Katz walked through the main entrance hall to get to the car, which was a slightly longer route than was necessary. MacLeod wondered why they had taken such a circuitous route to the car park but understood when, in the university's lobby, Professor Katz suddenly stopped both talking and walking, and smiled up at the stuffed likeness of the university's founder, Jeremy Bentham.

Bentham was a non-conformist who established the university in the nineteenth century. A utilitarian who continued to practise in death what he preached in life, he made provision in his will for his body to be dissected and his skeleton and head to be preserved. His stuffed, mummified carapace was then seated in his sedan chair and placed in the foyer of the university to encourage all visitors – especially non-conformists and dissenters – to reflect on his life's messages. MacLeod sensed that Professor Katz admired Jeremy Bentham and that it was part of his 'going home ritual' to contemplate the founder's remains as he left the university.

Professor and student sauntered out of the lobby and into the quad. The car was parked in front of University College London's classical pedimented portico, an imperial edifice set in front of a sweep of gravel and grass. There were just a few academics' cars parked in the quad – tatty, elderly, rusty and without grandeur or celebrity. Professor Katz walked over to his ancient Morris Minor, opened the door and sitting down, reached over to flick the lock, thus allowing MacLeod into the passenger seat. MacLeod, in a parody of Professor Katz's admiration for Bentham, admired the fine soft green paint of the car. He loved that particularly beautiful shade of Morris, and its matching darker green upholstery. MacLeod took his seat and looked around for a seatbelt, but there were none, as the manufacture of the car predated the change in the law that legislated for the compulsory wearing of seatbelts.

An expression of great concentration creased Professor Katz's face as he leaned into the steering wheel to start the car's engine. The car fired up easily and then lurched forward. Professor Katz hunched over the dashboard, cradling the steering wheel tightly in his hands. That lurch was odd, the car seemed underpowered, and MacLeod was puzzled at the peculiar reluctance and huge effort required to get the journey underway. The car almost stalled as it moved off, spluttering and straining as the gravel kicked up under spinning wheels. The Morris chugged through the entrance to University College without stopping and plunged into Gower Street, disregarding the oncoming rush of traffic. Professor Katz seemed unaware of the squealing of tyres and the angry beeping of the other drivers.

The Morris coasted forward in the stream of vehicles in Gower Street. Professor Katz stared benignly ahead, oblivious to the cars and buses that sped along around him. Professor Katz indicated right and an antique indicator flicked down from the window pillar. He then wound down the window and, risking amputation, stuck his arm out into the traffic indicating his wish to turn into Torrington Place. The engine raced and the Morris hiccoughed forward at 15mph.

Cars swerved to avoid the car but Professor Katz paid no attention to the drivers around him as he warmed to the theme of the earlier tutorial. Professor Katz's monologue continued along Torrington Place and then into Tottenham Court Road, where the professor waved his left hand to emphasise scientific points of interest. He held scant regard for the traffic lights at the Euston Road, and the Morris at full revs roared uncomfortably along the road until Professor Katz stopped at the junction of Hampstead Road and Drummond Street with his left foot, MacLeod noticed, on both the clutch and the brake pedals.

The traffic lights changed and the car jerked uncomfortably forward as Professor Katz revved the engine and released both brake and clutch. The Morris remained in second gear as they drove north, a puzzle to MacLeod who as they entered Camden High Street, was dying to ask Professor Katz why he hadn't ventured to use the full range of the Morris's gear box. Professor Katz's progress was erratic; his concentration was focused on the wonders of nerve conduction rather than on the glories of Camden Road. His eyes were mostly on his conversationalist with only occasional moments spent glancing ahead.

Eventually they arrived at their destination. Professor Katz drove in to a capacious parking space and the Morris juddered to a halt and then stalled.

MacLeod got out of the car and hurried around to open the door for his professor, still bursting to ask Professor Katz about his driving technique, and as the professor got out of the car, MacLeod enquired,

'Forgive me for asking, Professor Katz, but why is it that you stay in second and don't seem to change up or down gears?'

'Ach, MacLeod. It works well in second gear. I did try the other gears several years ago when I'd just bought the car. But you see there isn't enough power in third and fourth to take the car forward, and if I leave the car in second gear then I can travel quite satisfactorily without a problem.'

'But, Professor, what happens if you need to reverse?'

And the response came:

'My dear fellow, I've not needed to reverse.'

* * *

MacLeod's next contact with a famous scientist was in his final year at medical school. In a final year packed with exams, medical students are allowed an 'elective period' when they spend time away from their own medical school obtaining practical experience of medicine elsewhere in foreign parts. In these periods, some students travel to exotic places like Birmingham and Bradford but others go abroad.

MacLeod chose to go on his elective period to Stanford University in Palo Alto, Northern California. After the rigors of study and the intense period of swotting and exams, MacLeod wanted a rest in an easy-going environment where English was spoken and it was warm. Stanford ticked most of the boxes for him: the location was tropical and the natives did speak a variant of English.

He found the campus to be idyllic, gentle, warm and green. Everywhere there were bicycles. All around there were students. And there were marvellous birds, flashes of flying colour that were missing from the muted coats of English avian life: at Stanford even the blackbirds had red feathers. MacLeod hired a bike to get around. Cycling through the campus, he was amused by the university's architecture, designed in his view as an elaborate and costly joke. The campus buildings had a common architectural theme – the Mexican adobe hut. This worked well for the smaller buildings but failed empirically when the theme was used in the creation of a 50,000-seat sports stadium.

At Stanford, MacLeod's student life had a regular pattern. Every morning he would emerge from his lodgings, cycle through the streets of Palo Alto, lock up his bike outside the paediatric building and climb the stairs to the paediatric haematology wards, where he would meet his lugubriously competitive American medical student colleagues, all crew cuts and chinos – and that was just the women! The American students had been up on the wards since 4 am, just to get the edge. MacLeod greeted them at the beginning of his work day which was at a civilised 10 am, which in his opinion was a reasonable time to start the student day. The American students initially thought his late start most bizarre and tittered when he arrived at work, but then enlightenment dawned and they concluded that MacLeod's starting time was simply an expression of English work standards.

In the wards at Stanford, MacLeod learned a great deal about how medicine should not be practised. The British medical model worked on the principle 'First, do no harm', whereas the American model pivoted around the maxim

'First, give us your dosh'. MacLeod noticed how the American medical students' immediate response to passing their finals was to put a deposit down on a new Porsche.

MacLeod's antipathy towards American medical practice had been formed on a ward round in his first few days at Stanford. The round had begun outside an isolation room where a seven-year-old lingered awaiting a bone marrow transplant for leukaemia. In the corridor, the medical and nursing team faced the family. The father was drawn away from the entrance to the isolation room by the lead clinician. The discussion with the boy's father had not been about how well the child was doing with treatment or about the emotional aspects of his illness. Quite the opposite. The conversation between professor and father had been about the $150,000 cost of the bone marrow transplant. The father had not hesitated to say, 'We haven't the money, but that's OK, Doc. I'll mortgage the house.'

It was in this place, a blend of high academe and high profit, that MacLeod had spent a very pleasant couple of months, much of it by the pool, the rest of it drifting through the campus on his bike in his quest for the ultimate avocado sandwich. MacLeod felt that if he found this holy grail of bacon, bun and avocado, then his time at Stanford would not have been wasted. Interspersed between the bike rides and sandwich breaks, there were lectures and seminars, case conferences and ward rounds, all mildly entertaining, all intense, highly professional and learned.

At Stanford, there was no place for the diffident student, there to while away the time until the week prior to final examinations when seven days of furious cramming would serve its purpose of sufficiency, just enough knowledge to pass. At Stanford, there was a different way of studying compared to the model followed in the United Kingdom. Back home, anyone who studied was thought to be a swot. In Blighty, it was understood that it was only those students with insufficient mental capacity who needed to study. MacLeod observed the American students scurrying around the wards and libraries intent on their work: earnest, industrious, conscientious, competitive, selfish, driven, resolute and using whatever means they had to beat the other guy. The American medical students strove to be more successful, fought to achieve at a higher level than anyone else. With some amusement, MacLeod watched the students compete with each other. In exams, he observed pointers being moved on specimens, and slides knocked off microscopes as the Stanford students sought to sabotage each other's performances. For them, winning was all.

At Stanford, the lectures and seminars were given by world authorities, the diagnoses made on ward rounds were dazzling, everyone seemed so smart, so professional. And it was in this atmosphere of intense professionalism that MacLeod saw advertised on notice boards throughout the campus a poster that read,

'Denis Burkitt, Fellow of the Royal Society, visits Stanford'

Now Denis Burkitt was a magical figure, a demi-god in the medical heavenly pantheon. Dr Burkitt had trained as surgeon and then travelled to Africa where he was employed by the Ugandan Government, and he made many significant scientific observations whilst at work in Africa. His extraordinary skill was that he was able to link disease to their causes. In this capacity, he was one of those special medical scientists. His most important work had been to describe a cancer that affected young Africans and establish how the cancer originated. As a result that cancer now bears his name – the eponymous Burkitt's lymphoma. He drew maps of the geographical location of 'his' lymphoma and noticed that it occurred in areas of Africa where malaria was endemic. The mosquito, he surmised, was the carrier of the vector for the lymphoma. That vector was found to be a virus, the Epstein-Barr virus, which was identified by Professor Tony Epstein who had been inspired by Dr Burkitt's work to find the cause of the lymphoma.

Dr Burkitt's contribution did not stop at disease classification; he also designed treatments for the lymphoma, and his overview of disease and its origins continued beyond this. In later work, Burkitt described associations between diet and disease. He noticed that Africans living on their home continent had different patterns of illness to Europeans and Americans. And he observed that bowel cancer was unusual in Africa and common in industrialised countries. So Dr Burkitt theorised that a Western diet, rich in meat and low in vegetables and fruit was the cause of bowel cancer. High-fibre African diets are associated with large stools and short bowel transit time. Diets that are rich in proteins produce small stools with longer bowel transit times. Dr Burkitt surmised that the cause for colorectal cancer was the longer exposure of the bowel lining to the greater amount of toxins produced by the digestion of meats contained in a Western style as compared with a rural African-style diet.

So, MacLeod was very excited to see that one of his heroes was going to be at Stanford attending rounds and providing a commentary on presentations from the staff. A teaching round had been organised with an open invitation for all to attend. The meeting was to be held in the largest, biggest and most high-tech of all the lecture theatres on campus – a lecture theatre built on the adobe mud hut theme, of course. The rounds were ticketed and MacLeod made sure that he was amongst the first to book his place at the meeting. The seats were numbered and the best places were issued on a first come, first served basis. In due course, the ticket for the meeting arrived in his pigeonhole at the medical school. He opened the envelope and gloated over the ticket.

'How exciting!' he thought.

MacLeod's seat was in the third row. It was quite a coup to have got such a good seat, a place near the academic gods. He hoped to bask in the warmth of their presence and maybe catch something from the air that they exhaled. It was an unlikely prospect but possibly his best chance for future academic promotion.

The days went by, night following day, as is usual even in California! Days of idyll, nights of balm, days in the hospital, nights mostly alone because the students were so terrifyingly unfriendly, focused entirely on work and personal advancement. During the day, there was hardly a soul to talk to and

MacLeod's conversations were with the patients that he clerked, and the checkout counter staff at the supermarkets, where an abundance of supersize produce, brilliant red apples and enormous steaks, was packed into small brown paper bags that were destined to burst. In the evenings, MacLeod would walk through suburban Palo Alto. The houses were laid out in a typically American grid pattern, large single-storey buildings with lawns leading down to sidewalk and road. The grid system was a puzzle and MacLeod had no idea how the numbering of the houses was designated. The sprinklers were on and the air was loaded with a heady mix of barbecued meat and honeysuckle.

Two weeks passed and the day of the teaching round arrived. MacLeod thought that he should get to the session early. He knew that in the competitive world that is American medicine, his place might be snatched from him by a pushy student keen to ingratiate himself with the hospital hierarchy. MacLeod walked from the entrance of the lecture theatre complex to the steeply banked main lecture theatre, clattering down the stairs to his place in the 'stalls'. The theatre gradually filled up. Within a few minutes every seat was taken, but the flow of spectators entering the hall continued and the stairs became packed with people keen to listen to the great man.

In front of MacLeod, there was a single row of vacant seats, seats awaiting the arrival of the great and possibly good. A young doctor, whom MacLeod recognised from the wards as a particularly unpleasant research fellow, a man whose worm-like obsequiousness would have made Uriah Heap seem like Winston Churchill, took his place at the lectern, where he draped himself around the lectern, clinging to it for security.

Suddenly a door at the front of the lecture theatre pushed open and a line of dignitaries in academic gowns swept in. The waiting crowd hushed. A tall man whom MacLeod recognised as the Dean of Medicine, and the Head of the Hematology Department led the group in to the room. Their footsteps were loud; they were all male. They were all tall, all tanned and all fit, all of the same type and style, all of the same mould, except for one man, whom MacLeod recognised as Dr Burkitt. Dr Burkitt was ten inches shorter than the others, about two stones heavier and had no academic cloak. He wore a dark, unpressed, waistcoated suit, a suit of heavy wool that was completely unsuitable for Californian weather, a suit that was liberally decorated with food stains. Dr Burkitt's face was round and jolly; grey hair flopped in a characteristically British way over his brow.

The theatre lights dimmed as the dignitaries took their seats. The grim nerd from the dark lagoon swayed anxiously over the lectern. The first slide flickered on and suddenly the nerd was off hectoring the audience in a nasal drone as he described the 'case' of a poor child with Burkitt's lymphoma. The presentation style was characteristically intense, the story that unfolded heartbreaking, and the exposition of all of the scientific studies elucidating the biology of the child's lymphoma was of great depth and perception. The presentation for the esteemed visitor did justice to the enormous laboratory resources open to a great hospital based in an extraordinary university. The technology described was truly amazing and the treatment given was, of course, successful.

The lights were down low in a warm lecture theatre so that the projected slides could be clearly viewed, and as the slide show continued, the students could be seen leaning forward in their seats scribbling in their note books, not wanting to miss a single point of the presentation. About seven minutes into the presentation, MacLeod's attention was drawn towards the front of the lecture theatre, and more specifically to a repetitive dull sound that seemed to be billowing from the centre of the first row of seats. He was transfixed by the noise.

MacLeod then observed Dr Burkitt, slumped in the middle of the front row, abutted by the broad shouldered, and wedged into his seat by those shoulders. After eight minutes, Dr Burkitt's head lolled on to his chest. His neck flexed and MacLeod had a view of the rolls of flesh that tumbled over Dr Burkitt's collar. After nine minutes, Dr Burkitt hiccoughed forward in his chair but was prevented from rolling off his seat by the dean and the head of department who in the interest of politeness were pretending not to have noticed that, lulled by warmth, cosseted by darkness, soothed by the gentle tenor of the presentation, stupefied by the intensity of the science, Dr Burkitt, their esteemed guest, had fallen asleep.

The vibration of gentle snoring rumbled through the lower reaches of the lecture theatre as the speaker trawled through the pages of his presentation. But the audience was oblivious to Dr Burkitt's snoring, hardly noticing the ripples of sound, intent only on the content of the lecture. Slide after slide was projected to the audience and enthusiastic students raced to copy the outline of the talk into their note books. It was a tiptop talk, encrusted with learning, enamelled with information. It was a talk that was a credit to American medicine, a career-enhancing move for the presenter, and a glittering embellishment of Stanford's academic crown. It was a talk that Dr Burkitt seemed to be taking advantage of, too. Dr Burkitt, MacLeod noticed, seemed to be enjoying the talk in the depths of his dreams, and from time to time a flicker of a smile broke the calm of the great man's face. Dr Burkitt's lips mouthed the occasional word, echoing the presenter's speech and his belly rose and fell beneath his gravy-stiffened, partly buttoned waistcoat.

The Dean and the Head of Department paid no attention to Dr Burkitt's snoring. They stared straight ahead, their scrutiny only for the projected slides, their attention entirely devoted to the speaker. The Dean shifted in his seat and Dr Burkitt, losing purchase, slid forward in his seat. The strain on his knees as they bent beneath him forced him awake for a moment and with a

'Harrumph ...'

Dr Burkitt pushed himself back into his chair without opening his eyes. Wedged between the Dean and the Head of Hematology, he spent the next forty-five minutes of the talk in contented slumber. His breathing was regular, his eyes were closed. He was comfortable and cosy, stretched out on his seat in the front row of the lecture theatre with plenty of leg room.

The lecture spiralled to a spectacular climax with a denouement of the molecular changes thought to be involved in the viral oncogenesis observed in Burkitt's lymphoma. The lecturer turned to face the audience and ponderously closed his lecture notes to emphasise that his presentation had ended. The slide projector was switched off and the theatre lights were turned full on. The audience applauded the speaker and a rainstorm of decorous clapping filled the auditorium. The lecturer smiled. It was a complacent smile; a smug and self-satisfied smile that all but said,

'Thanks for the applause, and yes I do know it was a dammed good talk. But hey guys, applause is cheap. Where are the floral tributes?'

The Dean stood up to chair a question and answer session. He marched ponderously to the front of the lecture theatre. Back straight, head up, he stood centre stage and turned to confront his audience. In the absence of the Dean, Dr Burkitt slipped forward again and twisted out of his seat, knees bent, bottom bumping on the floor. Dr Burkitt woke with a jolt, and heavy with dreams, shook his head and seemed disorientated. He pushed himself up back on his seat.

Nobody seemed to notice him. All eyes were focused on the Dean who continued clapping while the audience followed his lead. Then the Dean stopped the applause and nodded commandingly at the audience. The audience hushed. The Dean walked forward a few paces and congratulated the speaker on an excellent presentation. Then he paced back, just two steps and then forwards, just two steps, so that within four paces there had been movement but little change in position. MacLeod considered the Dean's footsteps and realised that it was an attempt to intimidate the crowd. MacLeod waited for the Dean to begin the discussion with a question on the nature of the information that had been delivered. But MacLeod was wrong; the Dean had no intention whatsoever of leading the questions. Instead, he marched forward and smiling in Dr Burkitt's general direction, said in a voice redolent with pomposity, a complacent voice, a voice fat with the glory of medicine,

'Many of you in the audience will be aware of the incredible scientific importance of the work of Dr Burkitt. It is a great pleasure for me to welcome Dr Burkitt to Stanford on behalf of the faculty of medicine. It is, of course, a measure of the importance of Stanford that we are able to invite medical heroes and geniuses such as Dr Burkitt.'

The Dean turned to Dr Burkitt and continued,

'Dr Burkitt, may I sincerely say that it is a real honour for me to be able to welcome you to Stanford. We have listened to a really fascinating talk today. I wondered if you would like to deliver a commentary on this afternoon's presentation?'

MacLeod noticed that Dr Burkitt, having rubbed sleep from his eyes, was now pulling out a voluminous blue polkadot handkerchief from his pocket. Dr Burkitt, MacLeod concluded, had not heard the Dean's question.

'**Dr Burkitt**,' the Dean continued in a louder voice, '**would you like to comment on the case presentation?**'

Dr Burkitt sat up stiffly and shuffling in his chair stared in a surprised manner at the Dean. He seemed completely lost. Dazzled by the lecture theatre's lights, he rubbed his eyes again and then shook his head as if to orientate himself.

Dr Burkitt blew his nose loudly and stuffed the handkerchief back into his top pocket. He looked around the lecture theatre and seemed not to recognise his surroundings. He coughed and then settled back in his chair. He stared at the Dean as if he didn't know who the heck the man was. The Dean stared back at Dr Burkitt and waved his right hand in a limp circle that encouraged Dr Burkitt to respond to his question. But Dr Burkitt, still heady with sleep, thought that the Dean was addressing someone sitting a few rows back and turned to survey the packed seats behind him. He was greeted by puzzled stares and he turned back to the Dean and, smiling benignly, stuttered,

'Sssso sorry, old boy. What was that you said?'

The Dean smiled and with a wave of his hand to the audience, said, 'I wondered Dr Burkitt if you'd like to lead the discussion on the presentation.' The Dean bowed towards Dr Burkitt in recognition of the prestige granted to the institution by the presence of such an important guest. 'It's a great honour for us that you are here today.'

The audience hushed, waiting for Dr Burkitt's commentary to begin. But Dr Burkitt appeared confused. He wiped his brow with his left hand and seemed anxious. He looked around the lecture theatre for clues, but there were none to be had. The audience held its breath and Dr Burkitt muttered,

'I'm terribly sorry, but I was asleep.' His voice grew stronger, and he continued,

'Sorry, old boy. I missed the whole thing except for a few words at the beginning. Nice coffee and doughnuts though before the talk. Yes,' and Dr Burkitt became animated, 'many thanks for the doughnuts.

'Yes, that's right. Thanks for the doughnuts. That's what I wanted to say. Awfully good of you. Oh, and by the way – sorry I missed the talk. Fell asleep. Extraordinary! Don't know how it happened. I'm sure that the lecture was just excellent, though. They usually are. Goodness me, I slept right through it. Jolly good doughnuts, though. Thanks awfully.'

At that moment, MacLeod was the only member of the audience to laugh and in future times he would always treasure those words, simple words that deflated the self-importance and grandiose pomposity of the presentation and put into context the relative importance of doughnuts and medical lectures.

Chapter 5
Life Classes

MacLeod and ten jejune contemporaries gathered around the bed of a real patient. It was a person and it was breathing! It was not a pharmacology textbook; it was an actual patient, a woman of maturity and fascination. She held her sheets low over her bosom but not so low as to be indecorous or so high as to disguise the beauty beneath the sheets. Her eyes twinkled and her lashes were long. She looked at the medical students with interest and that interest was mostly for the boys.

Dr Owen had taken charge of the teaching round. He was senior registrar on the professorial medical firm. Dr Owen had a certain elegance and a definite style, and an air of knowledge and precision that inspired awe in the medical students. How could they hope to know as much as he knew? How could they ever be as he was? Dr Owen's white coat was immaculately laundered and fell around his knees in a beautifully starched sweep. His collar curled up to kiss his beautifully cut brown hair. His stethoscope was draped around his neck and placed so delicately that there was a perfect symmetry to the way it fell over his lapels. Dr Owen looked like a doctor in specialist training for an extensive private practice. When he smiled, the conversationalist blessed by his smile would catch a glimpse of seemingly perfect teeth, though the gleaming whiteness was set off by a hint of gold fillings.

'Now, gentlemen …' said Dr Owen – and the female medical students bristled.

J. Waxman, *MacLeod's Introduction to Medicine*,   57
DOI 10.1007/978-1-4471-4522-6_5,
© Springer-Verlag London 2014

'I want one of you to examine Mrs Judson's peripheries and then I will ask another student to move forward from the periphery to concentrate on an examination of the abdomen. Have you understood, gentlemen?'

Dr Owen nodded at Mrs Judson and motioned to one of the female medical students, who had apparently been designated a male for the afternoon, to attend to Mrs Judson's hands.

The student smiled anxiously at Mrs Judson and then at Dr Owen.

'Good start,' said Dr Owen encouragingly. 'Nice smile. Do go ahead, dear.'

'… emmm?'

'We are gathered together today as Englishmen on this ward round and I would encourage you, Madam, to converse in the language of this fair land, which is … English.'

The medical student stuttered and tears trickled down her cheeks.

'Take up Mrs Judson's hand, woman, and examine it. I have advised that you examine the periphery first. When I say periphery, I mean periphery. There is nothing more peripheral to the body than the hands, and in some instances, and we will consider this in a moment – the feet. Take Mrs Judson's wretched hand and examine it, you dolt.'

The medical student turned to Mrs Judson and took her hand. She turned the hand over and examined the palm and then the fingernails. Dr Owen watched the examination with interest.

'Perfect, perfect. And do you see anything worthy of attention in the hands?'

From the medical student, there came no answer to this question.

Dr Owen sighed and pulling up his trouser leg so that the material would not crease, bent at the knee and placed an exquisitely polished brown brogue shoe, size nine, on the edge of Mrs Judson's bed. He leaned forward and rested an elbow on his knee.

'Yes, dear. Is there anything that you've observed in Mrs Judson's hands that you'd like to comment on? Have you spotted anything gross?'

The medical student shook her head and let Mrs Judson's hand fall limply back on to the bed.

'Now, dear, tell me if you would, what exactly it is that you are looking for when you examine the hands?'

The medical student had no idea whatsoever. Dr Owen shook his head mournfully and a lock of hair fell over his eyes. He flicked this back and sighed.

'One is looking for clubbing of the fingers, one is looking for anaemia, one might be alert for signs of alcoholism, for cyanosis, the stigmata of ...'

Dr Owen's voice faded away, lost in ennui, he was tiring of the medical students before him. He glanced at his own nails and then pronounced laconically,

'Next!' No student rushed forward. '**Next student.**'

Next student shuffled up and his colleague scurried around to the end of the bed. Next student smiled at Mrs Judson who gleamed at him, straightened her nightdress and fussed with her hair.

'What can you see?'

The student took Mrs Judson's hand in his and blushed.

'Not much, Sir.'

'Not much? You can see her hand, can't you?'

'Yes, Sir.'

'Now, I have explained to your colleague that there are a number of signs that one looks for in the hands of a patient. You were listening, weren't you? You haven't been afflicted by sudden deafness syndrome, have you? And may I assume that you have not yet reached that stage of life when memory atrophies? Have you reached that stage? And I trust that you are not suffering at this moment from the depravities of a life of sin, such that your antics of the last twenty-four hours have deprived you of reason? Well? Answer? What do you see in this lady's peripheries?'

The medical student shuffled uncomfortably. He had continued to hold Mrs Judson's hand and, in his discomfort, was absentmindedly stroking her palm. Mrs Judson smiled radiantly and looked at the medical student with great interest.

'Oh, do put it down. And go away. Get out of my sight. You are hopeless. Next. I said **next**.'

The next medical student shuffled along and took up Mrs Judson's hand.

'Oh goodness! I have tired of you medical students. Enough of hands! On to the feet immediately.'

Dr Owen scowled at Mrs Judson.

'Are you decent, Madam?'

Mrs Judson nodded coquettishly and Dr Owen swept off her bedcovers to reveal Mrs Judson and Mrs Judson's fluffy, pink nylon, baby doll nightie. Mrs Judson's feet curled around each other for company. She simpered at the new medical student and fluttered her eyelashes at him outrageously.

The medical students stared at Mrs Judson revealed, Mrs Judson exposed, whilst the exposed and revealed Mrs Judson smiled at them all, and laid a hand on her chest in a gesture that appeared to be protective and modest but was in reality designed to emphasise the curve of her magnificent bosom.

Dr Owen marched to the head of the bed and scowled at the medical students.

'I want you to take a good look at Mrs Judson's feet, and then, gentlemen, we will proceed into the ward side room for a discussion. I take it that you are all looking at her feet? **The feet, you idiots! Look at the woman's feet!**'

Dr Owen looked disdainfully around the group of cowering students, and if the truth were to be told, then that truth was those who had more sheltered lives than their peers were, indeed, not paying much attention to Mrs Judson's feet. They were, in fact, also ignoring her hands and paying attention instead to the lustful curves of Mrs Judson's amorous bosom.

'The side room, gentlemen; gentlemen, the side room.'

Dr Owen swept away from the bedside and marching off the ward took up residence in the most comfortable armchair in the patient's sitting room which he had designated as the side room. There were two elderly ladies already sitting in the room.

Dr Owen glared at the ladies, but they paid no attention to his scowl. He rose from his chair as the medical students entered the room and stamped over to where the two patients were sitting. Towering over them he sneered, 'You may go'. The ladies hesitated and looked around to see who exactly it was that Dr Owen was addressing. Dr Owen made it clear that he was addressing them by courteously yelling,

'GO! GO AWAY! **SHOO!** GET OUT, **GET OUT!**'

Clasping their nylon dressing gowns to their necks, the poor old dears scurried out of the patients' sitting room. With a sidelong glance, Dr Owen watched their shadows disappear and turned to the students as they clustered around him.

'Not so close, move away from me.'

Dr Owen sat down in an armchair and, crossing his legs, exposed red silk socks. Then, lowering his voice conspiratorially, he asked,

'What do you think?'

Dr Owen sat back in his chair and surveyed the medical students disdainfully. MacLeod and his colleagues didn't know what to think.

'Answer me, you idiots!' Dr Owen screeched. 'Are you mute or are you just stupid?'

One of the students coughed and raised his hand.

'Well. What is it? Has someone put a penny in your slot?'

'It was a pound coin actually Dr Owen.'

'Cheeky. I like it.' Dr Owen swept back his hair from his forehead.

'You ask us what we think ...'

'Ah, an Oxbridge graduate, are you?'

'No, Sir, but if I could ask you, please? What we are meant to be thinking about, Sir? What is the question?'

'Good. I am delighted that one of you at least has some sense. I am asking you, gentlemen, about the lady's toenails.'

'The toenails, Sir?'

'Yes, man. The toenails.'

The medical student paused for thought.

'I am extremely sorry, Dr Owen, but I really don't understand your point.'

Dr Owen glowered at the student.

'The toenails were painted. You, Sir, have clearly led a sheltered life. Let this be your first clinical lesson. Beware the painted toenail, for painted toenails signify a dissolute life. The lady – and I use the term loosely – has painted toenails and this you must learn from me. If you learn nothing else in your preclinical lives, you must learn that a woman with painted toenails drinks gin in her bath. That will be all. You are dismissed.'

Dr Owen rose majestically from his chair and processed from the room. MacLeod was left with the feeling that Dr Owen's exit would have benefited from the presence of a mace bearer.

That evening MacLeod went with friends to a party in Southeast London. They drove to the party in Willie Nielsen's Ford Cortina, an antique with value, but an antique in need of such extensive restoration that its value was minimal. The party was in student digs in Deptford.

'Nice part of the world,' thought MacLeod, as they drove through high-rise council block canyons past a tumulus of burnt-out cars abandoned on the roadside.

'The party's great.'

MacLeod stood with his back to a table laden with French bread, brie, liver sausage pâté and bottles of Black Tower wine. The paper plates had run out and there was no cutlery. But this didn't prevent the party people from helping themselves to the grub.

Willie was keeping sober as he was the designated driver for the night. But the party *was* fun. The medical students conferred and agreed after a deep discussion that meandered between philosophy, casuistry and politics, that 'The women look fabulous!'.

And they did look fabulous in their bright-coloured tights and short dresses and, although MacLeod was too shy to dare to speak to girls, he was immensely cheered by the thought that one day he might. The party was very crowded. People danced wedged into each other; slow dancing to Grace Slick and Jefferson Airplane; slow dancing, but who would want to boogaloo to Jefferson Airplane? Pâté and brie, Black Tower and the *Dark Side of the Moon* – it was standard party fare.

At 2 am, it was time to go home and the boys piled into Willie's car. Willie was sober, absolutely sober. Turning to survey his raucous back-seat passengers, he grinned as he started the engine.

'Let's go, guys.' And they drove off along the New Cross Road.

The moon was high over Deptford and the stars were shining over London's night life. The road was relatively clear as it was so late. The initial part of their journey home was uneventful, the even rumble of the road broken by the hoots and shrieks of the medical students rollicking in the back of the car, ballooning with laughter, swigging from tall, black, dimpled bottles of cheap German wine stolen from the party. Each of the back-seat boys took their turn to recount tales of this or that night-time delight. And egged on, the stories became more and more elaborate, tales of conquest and debauchery spiralling into worlds of mischief, exaggeration and disbelief.

Leaving Deptford, MacLeod noticed a police car lurking in a side turning and at the moment that he noticed the police, the police noticed Willie Nielsen's Cortina and its back seat of riotous medical students.

The police car slid from the turning, like a toothsome shark, creeping up silently on its prey. The car kept them company for a mile or so and the noise in the back seat blossomed and bloomed. Willie was driving like a priest in charge of a tractor, both hands on the wheel, quiet, attentive, his route his guide. The police car drew closer and the shark opened its mouth. The back-seat boys bounced up and down and changed places in search of better positions in life. The neon lights of the twenty-four hour shops shone out on their journey and the traffic lights on green ushered them on their pathway home.

'All right in the back, boys?' And Willie looking in the rear-view mirror grinned at his pals.

It was unusual for Willie to be so stolid, so sober, so restrained. He was a fun boy and there was always some scheme for entertainment lodged in the dominant hemispheres of his brain and that scheme was usually expressed. Willie had a reputation which he took some pains to maintain. The 'giant's footsteps' were the apotheosis of his reputation, and on the building-block foundations of these footsteps Willie was happy to let his reputation rest. It was alleged that Willie had been responsible for the white-paint giant footsteps that traced a path up the side of the nurses' home. These footsteps tracked along a drainpipe to the fifth floor, they then took a sharp turn to the right as they reached the eaves and from there they continued horizontally, tracing the route of the gutters until they reached Adelaide Jones's bedroom window; and Adelaide Jones was a popular nurse. There, on the fifth floor of the nurses' home, at the fifth window from the corner, the footsteps stepped onto her window sill and entered her room. The footsteps had become a landmark, and gawping Japanese tourists formed queues to take pictures of the giant's progress.

Nobody had been able to work out how the footsteps had been painted on to the building. It would have taken a fireman's hoist to get the footsteps alongside the drainpipe all the way up from the basement boondocks to fifth-floor heaven, and this, it was rumoured, had been the way that the job was done.

But back to 2.20 am and to a certain purple Cortina, moss green growing in its window sills, a Cortina travelling westwards along the New Cross Road. It was the time of night when the London police did their utmost to enforce law and order. This they did by stopping for questioning every black man driving a new car in South London. But in Southeast London, the police were less selective – it was not only the black guys that they were after.

Meanwhile, as the police trailed the Cortina, the carousing in the back seat of the car entered its climax. The best of the Welsh element of the medical school rugby team was in good voice and the car's windows were wound down so that the neighbourhood could enjoy their harmonies.

Willie looked in the rear-view mirror again to check on his charges, and, as he did so, MacLeod saw Willie's benign smile change to a frown. MacLeod followed the direction of Willie's frown and looking round spotted that the police car had closed up on them and was now tailgating the Cortina. Willie's eyes narrowed. He was not fond of the police. His antipathy dated from an interview that he had been granted by the force, after a complaint had been made about the nurses' home footprints. There had been no charge but the lack of civility and good manners involved in the process had had a profound effect on young Willie Nielsen.

Suddenly Willie's driving style changed and, speeding up to just below the speed limit, he steered the car in towards the pavement and then out again to the white line in the centre of the road. He looked in his rear-view mirror at the police car which dropped back a few yards. It was clear that the police had their eyes on Willie's Cortina and they were waiting for an opportunity to stop the car. Willie slowed exaggeratedly and sped up again.

The approaching traffic lights turned amber then red and the Cortina came to a halt. The police car drew up behind the Cortina. The back-seat boys jumped up and down chortling and singing with a joie de vivre that would have been a credit to the Crazy Horse Saloon in Paris. MacLeod looked back at the police car and saw the concentration on the faces of the policemen as they scanned the Cortina for faults. He saw them staring with interest at the contents of the car and could tell that their intentions were not benign.

'Hey, Willie!'

'I know. The Filth are out to get us,' Willie whispered, his teeth clenched like Clint Eastwood on a night out in Mexico.

Willie revved the Cortina engine. MacLeod saw the police tense. Willie raced the engine and let off the clutch. The Cortina jumped forwards an inch. The police car inched forward, too, mirroring the Cortina movements.

'What are you doing, Willie?' MacLeod shrieked.

'Don't worry, MacLeod! Leave this to me.'

The back-seat boys, oblivious to the unfolding drama, sang more loudly and their harmonious intention was to raise the neighbourhood to virtue and religiosity. A bottle of Black Tower passed from hand to hand and then was accidentally dropped on the car floor. The police car's headlights flashed to full beam and the Cortina leaned alarmingly to one side as the medical students searched for the bottle of wine.

Willie revved the Cortina engine again. The lights were on red. The police car edged closer. Willie raced the engine.

'**Vroooom.**'

The police car driver hunched over his wheel.

The Cortina engine roared. Clutch off. The Cortina leaped forward three inches. The police car likewise thrust forward. Willie slammed on the brakes. He'd not crossed the line. The police driver hit his brakes, but not quickly enough to prevent the police Rover from smashing into the back of the Cortina. The lights were still on red and then they changed with the elegance of a ballet dancer, whirling through their sequence of red, red and amber, then green. Willie winked at MacLeod and turned off the engine. Meanwhile the back-seat boys, oblivious of the crash, continued singing, and it was a welcome in the valleys to all females locked in the Black Tower.

Willie got out of his car and walked to the police vehicle. The police driver lowered his window and looked out at Willie, who leaned in to the open window and stated the obvious,

'You've hit the back of my car.'

The police driver's face turned red. Apoplectic red. His eyes popped and bulged, and his mouth became a squashed winkle.

'I will need to take your details for my insurers,' said Willie.

Three policemen disentangled themselves from their seat belts and opening their car doors, put on their helmets and then surrounded Willie. In a gesture of friendship and loyalty,

MacLeod got out of the Cortina, squeezed through the circle of policemen and took his place next to Willie.

'Have you been drinking, Sir?' To which Willie, happily smiling, shook his head.

'Then you won't mind blowing into this would you, Sir?'

Willie puffed into the breathalyser. There was tangible disappointment on the officers' faces as they examined the breathalyser incredulously, passing it, one to the other, and shaking their heads.

'I will have to fill in an incident form.'

'That's OK," said Willie. "I guess I'll need that for insurance purposes, won't I, Officer?"

The policeman took off his helmet and scratched his head.

The mood was ecstatic in the Cortina on the rest of the journey home. Somewhere around Elephant and Castle, the giggling died down sufficiently for Willie to explain to MacLeod that, in law, the police were at fault for the crash because their car had run into the back of the Cortina. His car had been stationary at the time of the accident and the traffic lights had been on red. So Willie would end with a nice repair to the rusty rotten back end of his car. At this good news, the back-seat boys sang in praise of Jerusalem as Willie parked his car in the Principal's parking space in the medical school hostel's car park.

MacLeod found that life as a medical student might be serious at times ... but those serious times fell only in leap years. However, there was important work that had to be done, hours to be spent cramming for a seemingly unending series of endless exams, and it was perhaps out of a need for relief from all the studying that the bottled-up, pent-up, fed-up medical students so conscientiously exercised themselves in pursuit of the highest jinks. The students were told to smarten up for the ward teaching, and their costume changed to short white coats, no jeans, no beards, no earrings, no visible tattoos; they were scrubbed and brushed; garlic breath, sandals and ribaldry were all banned. They were to appear to be polite boys and girls, nicely brought up and ready to take their place as society's angels.

Their ward teaching was led by famous clinicians, headed by the portly waistcoats of Professor, the Lord Frankenstein, the Queen's physician, a great teacher, smiling on the fresh faces of yet another generation of apparent innocents as he explained about heart failure, aneurysms and anoxia. The lord was inspirational and charismatic, as all good lords should be.

MacLeod walked with his friends across Gower Street to University College Hospital for the afternoon clinical teaching session. They were to be taught the 'examination of the chest' by Professor Dent. The student group walked into the foyer of UCH and up the stairs to the first floor metabolic wards which were Professor Dent's domain and with Sister's permission ...

'Well, if you must ...'

... they gathered by the doors of the ward to await the arrival of the great man. They knew about Professor Dent and his work. He had described many of the biochemical process that regulated calcium metabolism and was famous for his meticulous studies in this area of medicine.

Professor Dent came on to the ward and nodded at the waiting students.

'Follow me.'

There was no welcome, there was no smile. Professor Dent seemed austere, cadaveric and cold, very thin and very pale, dressed in a British Home Stores' grey suit, scuffed black shoes and a curling collared yellowing white shirt: an academic without time to spare for clothes shopping. The professor stopped at the foot of a bed and stared at the patient huddled under the sheets.

'Good afternoon, Sir. These ...'

And he gestured weakly at the group of students,

'... are medical students. Would you mind if I taught them how to examine the chest? I believe the senior registrar asked you earlier? I take it that you won't mind? We do have your permission?'

The patient stared up from his bed at Professor Dent and MacLeod, looking at the poor man's face, saw a man thinner than Professor Dent, a man paler than the professor, a man more cadaveric than the professor. The patient raised his head from his pillow, and gasped,

'Certainly, Professor Dent. A pleasure, they've got to learn, haven't they?'

And with that, the patient's head dropped back on the pillow and he gasped for breath, exhausted by the effort of raising his head and talking.

The medical students had taken their places in a ring around the bed. They stood quietly and respectfully, in awe of the sober ascetism of the great man. Professor Dent positioned himself in the exact centre of the circle of students, hands clasped in front of him, a frown on his face. He surveyed the students and, when grimaced with distaste, MacLeod noticed that his teeth were yellowed and pointed. They were unsuitable teeth for a professor of medicine; they would have looked bad on a butcher!

'Today we are going to examine the chest. But before we do that, I should explain to you students that quiet observation is the key to diagnosis. A good doctor should be able to make a diagnosis without needing to do more than look at the patient. When you come to touch the patient, you do so, students, with a mind to proving the diagnosis that you have already made. Your hands are on his chest or his abdomen to find confirmation of the diagnosis that you have already established.'

There was something in the way that the professor spoke that drew all breath and light from the room. The ward had become airless and dark. His manner was portentous and severe. Arms crossed, face grim, no humour in the room, a priestly presence, a professor who was the highest acolyte of the god of learning, a man in search of the truth about calcium.

'Now, students, I am going to show you how to assess a patient's respiratory function. I gather that you have not examined the chest before, so I will show you all how to do this and hopefully set you on the right course for your future in medicine.'

MacLeod looked from the professor to the patient, from the man at the foot of the bed to the man lying in the bed. He was struck by how poorly they both looked, but whereas the professor seemed to have quite a lively look to his apparent ill health, the patient seemed to be convincingly sickly. The patient's breath came fast and shallow, his lips were blue and his nostrils flared with each poor breath.

Professor Dent seemed oblivious to the man's state and hectored the students in an earnest exposition of the right way to examine a patient's chest.

Then Professor Dent stopped talking and, drawing himself up, placed his index finger to his lips. The medical students huddled closer together and mirroring Professor Dent's posture, held themselves straight, trying to appear professional. MacLeod, shoulder to shoulder with his friends, waited to be picked on; he'd learned in earlier clinical teaching sessions that medicine's lessons were imparted not through a gentle apprenticeship but through bullying. In retrospect, many years later, thinking about these lessons, he felt that actually, yes, in truth, this had been quite a good way to teach because the student who is embarrassed by ridicule never forgets the clinical point.

Professor Dent drifted out of his reverie, the finger dropped from his lips and he addressed Willie, the student standing closest to the head of the patient's bed.

'You, Sir!'

Willie started and looked wistfully at his colleagues hoping that the professor was addressing someone other than him.

'Yes, you, Sir! I would like you to start the proceedings. I know that this is the first time that you will have examined a chest …'

Now MacLeod knew more about Willie's social life than Professor Dent and doubted very much that the professor's clinical observation was founded in fact. Willie had always made a point of examining the chest!

'… so let me help you in your assessment. The first thing that you should do is observe the patient closely. And you should do so from the foot of the bed. Go to the foot of the bed and observe …'

Willie did as he was bid, lumbering around to the foot of the bed as the other medical students drew back to allow him a view.

'And what do you see?'

Willie was at a loss to know what it was he saw. The patient was hidden under the bed sheets. Willie was speechless.

'Now, Sir, you will need to have a proper view of the patient.'

Professor Dent strode around to the side of the bed and, asking the patient if he minded, drew back the sheets so that Willie could see the patient properly. He stared at Willie as Willie stared at the patient and shook his head.

'No, Sir, that's no good at all. You need to be able to assess Mr Green's respiratory rate and chest movements. Girls, please help Mr Green sit up. Put him at angle of forty-five degrees in the bed. Plump up his pillows and shift him back in the bed would you?'

MacLeod noted how Professor Dent had relegated the female medical students to a subservient role. He hadn't asked the boys to sit the patient upright. The 'girls' dragged Mr Green up the bed and adjusting the headrest and pillows manoeuvred him to an angle of precisely forty-five degrees to the horizontal. Professor Dent walked back to the foot of his bed and stood by Willie's side contemplating the patient's breathing.

'Help Mr Green off with his pyjama jacket, would you?'

The girls leaned Mr Green forward and helped him undress. The effort was exhausting for Mr Green and he collapsed back on his pillows breathing heavily, his eyes shut. Professor Dent looked disdainfully at Willie as he stared at Mr Green's chest.

'You will need to time his respiratory movements. You do have a watch with a second hand?'

Willie had no watch, and borrowed one from a colleague. He timed Mr Green's breathing.

'That's twenty-six breaths in a minute, Professor.'

'Correct. The normal number of breaths taken in a minute is around thirteen to fifteen, so you will see from your first observation that Mr Green is breathing rapidly and you will be thinking, of course, about the causes for his problem and these could range from chronic obstructive pulmonary disease to heart failure. Next student!'

Willie joined the circle of medical students and Professor Dent's next victim walked around to the foot of the bed. This time, the professor's prey was Colin Trask, an Oxford hockey Blue; he was tall with blond hair and a chin that pointed the way. Professor Dent smiled encouragingly at Colin. Professor Dent was President of the Hockey Club.

'Now, Sir, you will observe Mr Green's chest movements and see that he is using his accessory muscles of respiration. His sternomastoids are contracting and his abdominal muscles are tensing. This will tell you that Mr Green is in respiratory distress.'

MacLeod observed that Mr Green was, indeed, in considerable respiratory distress. His head had lolled forward on his chest and his tongue was protruding from his mouth.

Colin nodded at the professor and was dismissed. It was now Emerald's turn to come to the foot of the bed and as she did so, Professor Dent hissed,

'Not there, girl; go to Mr Green's side. No, not that side, his right side. Patients are always examined from their right side. Take his hand in yours, there's a good girl, and tell me what you find.'

Emerald stuttered but all that came from her mouth were letters. There were no words.

'You will tell me, please, about the temperature of Mr Green's peripheries, the colour of his nails, whether a flap is present and give me a view please on his pulse.'

Emerald was transfixed; she had no idea what she should do.

Professor Dent walked around the bed and took Mr Green's hand in his. Mr Green's arm was quite limp and Professor Dent had to lift up his arm from the bed.

'You will see that he is cyanosed – his nail beds are blue, that he has palmar erythema – his palms are reddened, that he has a flap ...' and Professor Dent bent Mr Green's hand back at the wrist and MacLeod could see the rigidity and spasm that followed this movement,

'... and that his pulse is weak and irregularly irregular. These are signs of profound respiratory failure and atrial fibrillation. That will be all. Next student.'

Professor Dent glared at the next student who, unfortunately for him, was not a member of the Hockey Club.

'Examine the jugular venous pressure.'

The student started forward to his position by Mr Green's side and then stared at Mr Green's neck hoping for inspiration. At that point, Mr Green's head fell forward on to his chest and his breathing slowed.

'I can't make it out, Professor.'

'Look, boy. There it is. It's there. See? It's at the angle of the jaw. Can't you make out the JVP? If you've trouble seeing it, press on the patient's liver; press gently. No, not like that. Press gently, I said, and the JVP will rise with the pressure on the venous system. Now who's next? You, Sir. Yes you, Sir. Step forward.'

'We will now assess Mr Green's respiratory movements. This you do by placing your hands on the chest wall. You should put them on the chest wall as if your hands are the wings of a bird and observing your hands make an assessment of the amount of respiratory movement on both sides of the chest. You will be asking yourself, Sir, whether the chest movements are full or limited, and indeed whether they are equal or unequal. Next student.'

'You, girl. Yes you. I want you to percuss the chest. Like this. Your right index finger is a hammer falling on your left middle finger which is placed flat against the chest wall. You will inch forward with your hand, percussing the chest, and from the resonance beneath your finger will be able to tell whether there is consolidation, an effusion or normal lung below. Yes, like that. Good. Help Mr Green forward, would you, so that the girl can examine the back of his chest?'

Two sturdy medical students stood at either side of Mr Green's shoulders and heaved him upright so that the student could percuss his chest. Mr Green was limp in their arms. They held him forward and the student tapped out a dull plangent note, edging from the lung bases to the apices, conducted by Professor Dent with a wave of his hands.

'Excellent. Next student. You, Sir. Yes, you. Step forward, there's a good chap. You have a stethoscope, Sir?

'Good. Warm the bell of the stethoscope and then place it on Mr Green's chest. No, not like that. No. For goodness' sake, Sir! Do take the stethoscope and warm the end in your hand, there's a good chap. Thank you. Excellent! Well done! Now place the bell of the stethoscope on Mr Green's chest and edge the bell over the chest listening attentively to his breath sounds. You will need Mr Green to breathe through the open mouth – that way the sounds are loudest. Then, Sir, from the character of the breath sounds, you will be able to draw a conclusion as to the pathological process below.'

MacLeod looked with interest at the scene before him. Mr Green was leaning forward supported by two large medical students, one on either side of him. The poor man's breathing was irregular and noisy. His eyes were shut and his head hung forward, chin lodged on his chest. It was with an effort that the students managed to keep him upright. The student charged with examining Mr Green leaned over him, stethoscope clamped to the man's back.

'I can't hear a thing, Professor Dent.' The medical student, stethoscope lodged in his ears, bent his head towards Professor Dent, a look of puzzlement on his face. Professor Dent looked irritated.

'For heaven's sake, Sir! Aren't you capable of the most elementary task? Ask Mr Green to take big breaths in, you fool. Big breaths in through the open mouth.'

The student nodded.

'Big breaths in, please, Mr Green; through the open mouth, please.'

There was no response from Mr Green. Professor Dent exploded with irritation.

'Inspire, Mr Green!'

There was a flicker of recognition on Mr Green's face and MacLeod saw him take in a tiny breath. The medical student, stooped behind Mr Green's back, face buried in the patient's pillow, nodded; he'd heard the breath sounds. Professor Dent looked imperiously at the cast of students.

'There,' he said. 'If you say what you want the patient to do with confidence, then it is done.'

The medical student waited; he'd heard one breath sound and he wanted to hear more. He looked up at Professor Dent, expectantly. Professor Dent surveyed the scene, liked what he saw and said,

'... and expire.'

There was no response from the patient.

"Expire!" Professor Dent commanded.

With that, poor Mr Green collapsed back in the pillow, quite limp, head at an unpleasant angle on his chest, arms at rest on the sheets, toes turned in, breathless – and expired.

The medical students gasped, looked at Mr Green with panic and then turned to Professor Dent. Professor Dent's spectacles gleamed and sparkled, reflecting the ward lights. Then Professor Dent smiled enigmatically, his smile that of a barn owl surveying a fat mouse scurrying home through the fields.

The ward was silent, the medical students horror-struck. This was their first death. They'd seen nothing of death before. Mr Green was dead. Mr Green had done what Professor Dent had told him to do. Such was the power of a famous physician. The patient had expired on request.

Professor Dent straightened his tie, nodded at the medical students, and with a 'Good day to you all', walked from the bed towards the doors to the ward. The students saw him stop at the nurses' office, knock and, as the door opened, heard him say,

'Sister, could you see to Mr Green?'

Chapter 6
The Bed Jape

It was a gloomy winter afternoon and MacLeod was a bored prisoner, caught by the awfulness of yet another period on call when he could have been out in the wide world having fun. The day had drawn on as it almost invariably did with its prospect of unending work and a few moments of interrupted sleep in a bony bed. MacLeod disliked being on call almost as much as he disliked the hospital managers. And the thought of hospital managers brought him to the mumbling view that,

'They're a plague – a plague of parasites. I *hate* them. I *loathe* them; they're a barrel of infected idleness. Why are they here? There isn't a reason. They're useless, grossly over-paid and completely superfluous. Grrrrrh. And God they're ugly.'

To MacLeod and most of his colleagues, the managers seemed to have an unnecessary existence. They themselves defined their role and they seemed irrelevant to every aspect of health care. They had no place in any hospital. MacLeod just couldn't see the point to them.

'What do they do?' he mused, and 'Nothing!' was the answer that echoed back at him, though how nothing could have an echo was a puzzle to MacLeod and he mused about nothing's echo for a while.

But the managers' days were filled with activity of a sort. It was rumoured that the short hours that managers spent at work was usefully filled by the writing and circulating of

J. Waxman, *MacLeod's Introduction to Medicine*,
DOI 10.1007/978-1-4471-4522-6_6,
© Springer-Verlag London 2014

memos, memos that were posted into the internal mail and then delivered to adjacent third-floor managerial offices.

'But surely they must do other things, too?' one of MacLeod's pals had asked as an aside on a ward round, instead of checking a drug chart as the consultant had requested.

In the bar that night, they had voted Emerald onto the case. A couple of days later, she'd taken a day's holiday to spy on the managers and find out what exactly they did in their 'working' life when not memo writing.

The managers at University College Hospital occupied a single floor of the Private Patients' Wing, a wood-panelled corridor of comfortable offices on the third floor of a Victorian red-brick building. Emerald had wrapped up in a trench coat, dark glasses and a muffler, and armed herself with a camera, clipboard and a stopwatch. She installed herself under a lamppost and followed the managers as they emerged from their offices.

A meeting of the Doctors' Mess was held on the following day. Emerald, standing on a chair, called the reprobates to order with a claxon. She showed them the clipboard's evidence, and projected the photos that she'd taken onto a screen.

Emerald's sleuthing revealed that it was true that the managers were rarely seen beyond the third floor. She reported that when the managers emerged from their offices, they seemed to scurry, rather than walking normally, their eyes fixed on the floor to avoid contact with humanity – working humanity. Emerald suspected that the managers were concerned that any eye contact might lead to their being questioned as to the purpose of their outing or even their existence.

She'd told the meeting that she had actually stopped a couple of the managers, explained that she was doing a survey of street life for the Council, and asked them what they were doing out of their offices. And in reply they'd claimed that they were about to have a meeting about an important memo and had been 'tasked' with a rare and highly strategic mission, a voyage to the canteen to buy a sandwich. Emerald informed the packed meeting of the junior Doctors' Mess that when they weren't writing memos, the rest of the managers' working week was spent in the canteen. Emerald put to the group that her work had left her to suspect,

'... and this is entirely supposition ... that on some days this journey to the canteen might be the entirety of their measured output, as they'd written no memos.'

None of the medical staff had been inside the management offices which they imagined to be highly luxurious. But regardless of their state of decoration, the fact that the managers had offices whilst the doctors and nurses were not even allowed paper clips or filing cabinets, let alone offices, was indeed a matter for some comment.

During their time as students and then junior doctors, MacLeod and all of his friends had noticed that the numbers of administrative staff employed in hospitals had burgeoned. The history of this growth in the number of managers had started with the introduction of the internal market by the Thatcher Government. The internal market had been designed to introduce competition between hospitals. To facilitate this process, health treatments were priced and charges for services were introduced. Notional costs for hip replacements and pneumonias, cancer treatments and appendectomies were established. Bills for patients' treatments were then issued by hospitals to the patients' local health authority.

With time, the management structure of the NHS changed, and the health authorities were replaced by the Primary Care Trusts, and then by a stroke of amazing managerial genius, the bills got sent to the PCTs instead of the health authorities. This billing mechanism would, it was hoped, allow GPs to choose between hospitals, and buy their patients' treatment from the cheapest provider. But it was unclear to MacLeod and his colleagues how the internal market would produce any competition. This was because hospitals had arisen in geographical locales to fill a local need and it would be unlikely in the grand scheme of things that it would save money if patients were shipped to Leeds from London because hip surgery there was 10 % cheaper.

'Besides,' MacLeod wondered, 'had anyone ever considered the cost of producing and settling bills into the costs equation?'

In the view of many doctors, the expense involved in administering the billing system far outweighed any notional advantage of a 'free market' in health care.

The burden of administration on the NHS would become disproportionate over the years, as it grew unchecked and unregulated, transforming over the decades after Thatcher into a monstrous unaccountable hegemony, self-regulating and out of control. The levels of ignorance and stupidity, the lack of education and sensitivity, the arrogance and idiocy that the doctors, porters, nurses and medical secretaries were confronted with when they scrutinised the serried ranks of managers, was a cause for immense irritation and frustration. But should any doctor, porter, nurse or medical secretary point out that the administration was out of control, then the forces of evil would find focus and discharge venom on the poor complainant who found himself out of a job or with less salary than he had before the complaint because the managers were in charge of the annual individual meetings that led to the regulation of doctors' salaries.

But to return to MacLeod and his ricocheting mumbling. Within a few minutes, he'd worked out the details of a '**Plot Against Management**'. On that dark winter afternoon on duty in the hospital, MacLeod came to the conclusion that the time had come to point out to the managers the futility of their existence. MacLeod's sense of irritation, his feeling that the work of the managers was outrageously irrelevant, led him to plan a jape that would be fun; sport to occupy the hours of his imprisonment, righteous sport that would cheer up his fellow prisoners.

MacLeod knew that the managers' offices were cleaned at 6.30 in the evening. The cleaners could, of course, have chosen to clean any time after 4 pm or before 10.30 am because the managers never worked late nor started work early. MacLeod needed an accomplice for his adventures and chose a soppy sort of fellow who would go along with his plans. That fellow was Wilson. Some of Wilson's colleagues had wondered how he'd got into medical school but desisted from questioning him directly when they noticed that Wilson had a low centre of gravity and walked dragging his knuckles along the floor. Wilson played a robust game of rugby, had gone to an excellent public school, and his father was a cousin of the Dean – all excellent reasons for admission to medical school.

MacLeod bleeped Wilson and asked to meet him in the underground corridors of the hospital that connected the ward blocks with Casualty and the labs. As MacLeod explained his plan, Wilson backed against the corridor walls and anxiously checked his pager.

'What *we* are going to do,' MacLeod told Wilson, 'is some furniture arranging. OK?'

Wilson nodded his agreement. He liked furniture arranging, always had.

'But look, Wilson, the furniture arrangement is going to be a surprise for our colleagues. They know nothing of our plans. It's a surprise. It's a secret. So, shhhh ...' and MacLeod held his index fingers to his lips.

'Got that, Bonehead? It's secret. Now listen. Here's the first part of the plan. Before we do the furniture arranging, we have to secure access to some rooms. OK? You're not to worry now with the details. We'll meet up in thirty minutes. And keep the evening clear, Bonehead. Don't let the registrar bother you. If he wants to go round the patients, tell him he can go round by himself for once. And remember it's a secret. We mustn't let anyone else know anything about what we're doing. I'll see you around 6.30.'

Wilson nodded his agreement.

It seemed that the silly chap would agree to anything.

'See you later, Wilson. OK?'

So, at 6.30 pm precisely, MacLeod and Wilson skipped up the first two flights of stairs of the Private Patient's Wing of

University College Hospital, pausing only briefly to look through the windows and admire for a moment the fantastic giant white footsteps that Willie Nielsen had painted on either side of a drainpipe going up the wall of the nurses' home.

'Now that's what I call art,' said Wilson and MacLeod agreed.

In MacLeod's opinion, Willie's work out-conceptualised the whole body of conceptual art produced in the last century. It outclassed everything from Duchamp to just about everyone. It was a work of art worthy of any great gallery, a work that, in his view, should be considered by Tate Modern for their next purchase. And how amusing would that be if the Tate bought the back wall of the nurses' home. MacLeod imagined the effect of removing the whole of the back wall,

'Wouldn't that be great, particularly if it happened at bath time?'

MacLeod and Wilson proceeded carefully up from the second to the third floors. They sneaked along, stopping at the hint of a footstep, freezing at the rumour of an approaching person. As they reached the third-floor landing, they crept slowly around the lift shaft and bent double. They stooped down and leaned on each other, sinking low so that they could not be seen through the half glass doors that marked the entrance to the third-floor managers' offices. MacLeod peeked stealthily through the glass. It was 6.35 pm and the suite of administrative offices was being cleaned. Looking through the glass, MacLeod saw that there were three cleaners in the third-floor corridor, plump be-bucketed women in green uniforms – vacuum cleaners, mops and dusters, at the ready. The women were moving very slowly, they were somnambulists with dusters, an arthritic ballet of Jeyes fluid and Harpic.

MacLeod turned to Wilson, who stood up suddenly, awaiting instructions. MacLeod put fingers to his lips,

'Shush!' and gesturing frantically to him, whispered,

'Get down, you clown or they'll spot us.'

Wilson and MacLeod, on their knees behind the door, gradually raised their heads over the wooden door frame and peered at the cleaning ladies as they went about their tasks. The women had keys at their belts, third-floor chatelaines. MacLeod and Wilson watched the cleaners as they gradually shuffled along the corridor. They saw that as each woman approached an administrator's office they'd pause, scratch and then remembering what they're supposed to do, fumble for a key, insert it in the lock and turn the Yale to enter the room. The room door remained open whilst the cleaner vacuumed and tidied.

One of the women turned in their direction.

'Keep your head down, Bonehead! MacLeod whispered as he shoved Wilson's chin down below the door glass. 'Keep it down as low as you can. Listen, I'm going to sprint into that corridor as soon as the coast is clear. Your job is to let me know when all of the cleaners are in the managers' rooms. I'm going to be on my mark down here ready to rush in when you give me the word. Have you got it? Just let me know, right?'

Wilson grunted and raised his head just a little so that he could look into the corridor. He saw just one woman who was shuffling along to the far end, swinging a bucket. MacLeod pulled off his shoes.

'Now!' Wilson mumbled, 'She's gone in. Quick!'

And MacLeod, a partly unravelled roll of Sellotape stretched between his hands, pushed through the half glass door and into the managers' corridor. MacLeod padded along the floor in his socks, his movements resembling a parody of a drunken ostrich. At the first of the office doors, MacLeod turned to Wilson. He saw the idiot grin, the idiot nose slapped up against the glass, the idiot breath condensing on the pane; saw his pal and winked. Then, turning to the first of the office doors, MacLeod concentrated intently as he silently wrapped Sellotape around the Yale lock. MacLeod knew that when the door was closed by the cleaner, the Yale bolt would not secure the room. MacLeod turned to Wilson and winked again Wilson held his hands over his eyes in panic, not quite the alert scout that MacLeod needed at that moment to ensure his safety.

Suddenly the clatter and thump of heavy footsteps threatened to emerge from a room further along the corridor. MacLeod bolted for safety and pushed through the corridor doors. Panting slightly, MacLeod from the exercise, Wilson in sympathy, the pair crouched behind the corridor doors. A minute later, courage in hand, hand in pocket, they both stood up and peered over the edge of the glass into the corridor. One of the cleaners had come out of a manager's office and was scuffing along the corridor towards them, dragging her bucket and mop, water slopping onto the hallway floor carpet.

Wilson gasped. MacLeod shoved Wilson's head down.

'Quiet, keep quiet you fool. Get down you idiot. They haven't finished cleaning yet. For goodness' sake, Wilson! Don't panic, Bonehead.'

The thumping approached and their heads sunk lower. For a moment, MacLeod wondered if they were about to be discovered. But the shuffle of footsteps on corridor floorboards suddenly ceased and the tinkle of keys could be heard by the naughty pair.

'She's going into another room! Here's our chance!'

MacLeod pushed through the swing doors, unravelled Sellotape at the ready, and in a trice he had secured three more rooms. He turned to scamper back and saw Wilson staring at him through the glass panel, hands over his ears. MacLeod rushed back and the two dived to the floor again.

'Six more offices to go, Bonehead and then that's it.'

'What do you mean, "that's it"?'

'Well done, Bonehead! You're quite right, that's not quite it, but it will be it for now, as soon as I've done the other offices. Stand easy, Bonehead. We're about to complete Phase One of Black Ops. We're nearly "done", old buddy.'

MacLeod stared through the glass into the corridor as the cleaners emerged and entered offices. Seizing his moment, Sellotape at the ready, he pushed through the swing doors and, still in his socks, silently secured six more rooms.

'That's it, Bonehead. We're out of here before we get caught. See you later. OK?'

As midnight approached, MacLeod and Wilson reconvened as planned. They wandered through the runnels and tunnels that lay under the unhealthy mass of mortar and bricks, pus and piles that was UCH. MacLeod and Wilson stood at a corridor corner. MacLeod gazed at his watch. The seconds passed and Wilson stared at MacLeod staring at his watch. The silence was broken.

'Right, Bonehead. It's midnight. Time to roll, big boy.'

And at that point, precisely at the stroke of midnight, MacLeod and Wilson entered Phase Two of their mission. In the bright lit darkness, they giggled and gossiped as they skipped over the ruby red cockroaches that skittered through the hospital's basement corridors. They'd found some redundant hospital beds, unwanted and unused, retired from service and waiting for the scrapheap. MacLeod had come across them, piled in a forgotten corner and the sight of them had been the spark that ignited the flames of fury that consumed him. They wanted those beds, needed them to complete the little treat that they had in store for the managers. The beds had wheels, and the two men pushed them along, one by one to the lobby of the lift shaft at the basement of the Private Wing. Collecting all of the beds and rolling them on through the corridors was quite a task, but it was exhilarating and it was fun. After about twenty minutes of heaving and shoving, the job was done and MacLeod and Wilson contemplated the collection of beds lodged in the lift shaft lobby. MacLeod issued instructions.

'OK, Wilson, we'll only get one bed in the lift at a time. I'll go up first and check that the coast is clear. Then so long as all's clear, I'll send the lift down to you. Focus, Bonehead. Concentrate, right? This next bit is your part of the job. When the lift comes down, you're to push the first bed into the lift and send it up to the third floor. You hang on here, you're not to get into the lift. The lift is for the beds, not us. I'll send the lift down when I've taken out the bed and then you're to send the next one up to me on third floor. Got it? All beds to the third floor.'

Wilson nodded. MacLeod worried that the complexity of the intellectual skills required to count to two might be beyond Wilson's brain, but he was hopeful …

MacLeod bounced up the stairs to the third floor. He looked along the management corridor and there was no one in sight. The coast was clear.

As planned, MacLeod then sent the lift down to the basement and waited with some anxiety as the indicator registered the lift's descent and ascent. The lift door opened and he trundled the first of the beds out of the lift and pressed the basement level button again. He waited for a couple of minutes and then saw that the lift was once more on its way up.

'Good old Bonehead – he's got the hang of it!'

MacLeod heaved the bed from the lift and out into the corridor and then pressed the control button for the basement. He watched the lift doors shut and turned to push the bed through the swing doors that led from the lobby into the third floor corridor.

MacLeod waited by the lift. The moments passed by. The lift seemed fixed at the basement level. MacLeod waited, watching the lift indicator with some anxiety but his anxiety turned to relief as the lift indicator twinkled into life and showed the lift rising through the floors. It had been a tricky moment. Considering the situation as the lift climbed through the shaft, MacLeod came to the view that Wilson had probably forgotten how to count to three, but to give the man his due, he'd remembered eventually and so it would seem that the interviewers who had selected him for medical school had done a good job!

'Now that Bonehead has got the hang of counting to two he might have prospects,' MacLeod considered, 'of having a successful medical career.'

MacLeod mused that Wilson was clearly in possession of all of the requisite skills necessary to succeed in medicine. With his skill in counting to two and his enormous size, a career in orthopaedics was a possibility. The lift doors opened and MacLeod pulled out another bed. He pressed the button for the basement and this time went down with the lift and basted Wilson with encouragement,

'Keep up the good work, Bonehead. You are a star!'

There were now ten beds blocking the third-floor corridor and it was time to move those beds to their resting place. Wilson had come up to the third floor with the last of the beds. He stood in the lift lobby scratching his head. His shirt had unravelled from his trousers and his jaw hung open. Wilson stared at MacLeod as he approached the first of the office doors. MacLeod pulled the door open without resistance. As MacLeod had anticipated, the Yale hadn't done its job and secured the room because the Sellotape had prevented the Yale bolt from closing.

'OK, Wilson, let's go for it. On to Phase Three. Roll up a bed there's a good chap.'

The Bonehead did as he was told and obediently pushed a bed into the first administrator's office.

'Good man, Wilson. Now park it on the carpet and we'll move the desk out. Give me a hand with the stuff on the desk, would you.'

MacLeod and Wilson cleared the computer, telephone and files from the administrator's desk onto the floor and heaved the desk out into the corridor. They manoeuvred the bed into position next to the window, placing it exactly where the desk had been. And then they put the files and phone and computer on to the bed, positioning them so as to replicate their original location on the desk.

They stepped back to check that all was as it should be. MacLeod thoughtfully drew up the desk chair into position by the bed. Walking from the room, MacLeod yanked the Sellotape from the Yale. The bolt sprang back into place and the door closed with a soft click.

'Well done, Wilson, you are a good fellow and not half as dumb as people say. On to the next room, come along, there's a good fellow.'

The next room was a woman's office. There were flowers on the desk and a framed photograph of a husband and two small children, rosy-cheeked and very ugly replicons of the sperm donor.

'Out with the desk, Wilson. Well done!'

The desk was shuffled into the corridor, the bed moved into the office, desktop bibelots reassembled and it was off with the Sellotape and next office, please. In time, quite a good deal of time actually, the two junior doctors had converted all of the third-floor offices into dormitories, a droll statement they thought of the reality of the lifestyle and work ethic of the incumbents of the third floor of the Private Wing of University College Hospital.

And then it was time for Phase Four of the operation. There were around fifteen desks that had been piled into the third-floor corridor and these needed to be shifted down into the basement to the spot where the beds had been found. Moving the desks down into the basement corridor was quite a task. It was a good thing that Bonehead was a beefy rugby ace, otherwise the whole process would have been almost impossible. But bless him, Bonehead hadn't baulked. Rather the opposite! He rejoiced in the heavy work – this was extra training that would serve to bulk up his muscles and build warrior potential for the next scrum down.

At around 2.30 am, their task was completed. In the deepest corridor of the hospital, Doctors MacLeod and Wilson admired the collection of desks that occupied the basement bed repository. Although miraculously their bleeps hadn't gone off, the boys did their duty before turning in and sauntered to the wards to chat to their favourite nurses and, as an aside, check whether any of the patients needed sorting out. They surveyed a ward of snores and farts; the patients were looking good and so were their prospects for a peaceful night, the deserved reward of the righteous and just. And so it was that MacLeod and Wilson went off to bed contented and tired, to the most profound of sleeps, entered into with the deepest sense of satisfaction and fulfilment that naturally springs from a job well done.

Morning came and at 8.30 am both of the boys were on ward rounds, rounds that ricocheted through shared wards.

And when the rounds collided, Wilson and MacLeod smirked, catching each other's glances. They expected no incriminations until later in the day, when the managers arrived at work.

MacLeod's ward round was with his surgical consultant, Mr Cowie, whilst Bonehead, most appropriately – given his skills as a rugby player – was on rounds with the orthopaedic consultant, Mr Bailey. The orthopaedic rounds ignored the patients and concentrated on the carpentry, the consultant and senior registrar gloating over the accuracy and depth of nail insertions, enjoying the hidden beauty of shiny titanium prostheses. At the end of the surgical and orthopaedic rounds, the two consultants and their staff collided in Sister's office on ward 1.3. The consultants sat down with tea and biscuits with Sister, whilst the registrars and housemen stood with tea and no biscuits.

Pleasantries were exchanged between the consultants.

'Remember old Muffin?'

'Of course, old boy! How could one forget Muffin?'

'No, not that Muffin, not Muffin the Mule, I mean Muffin the fool.'

'That's just the chap I was thinking of. Fine fellow. Good chap.'

'Absolutely. He's doing very well you know.'

'Harley Street?'

'No! Surprising really. In prison actually. Fiddled the books. After medical school, he went into private general practice in Wimpole Street. Seemed to be doing very well, nice car, nice wifey, etc. But – and this is the point – it was all a bit of a sham.'

'What do you mean, old boy, was the wifey really a chap? I thought he was a bit odd when he was at medical school with us. Used to wear a blue blazer. Very unconventional. Damned unconventional, I'd say.'

Wilson and MacLeod looked at one other over the rims of their teacups and winked. One of the registrars' bleeps went off and he left the room to answer it.

'No, it wasn't that he was a queer or anything like that. It was far less serious. Old Muffin made all sorts of fictitious claims to the private insurers. Claimed that he had carried out various medical procedures. But, of course, he hadn't! Chap wasn't capable of that sort of work. You remember him don't you?'

'Course I do. I remember old Muffin. Wasn't capable of darning a sock, never mind writing a prescription. How did the fellow qualify?'

'Qualify? They took pity on him at his third and final attempt. Anyway, as I was saying, old boy, the chap made claims for medical procedures that he hadn't actually carried out.'

'My dear fellow, that's hardly a crime. Surely we all do a little of that, don't we?'

'Point is that he did it on rather a grand scale. Not the odd sixpence here and there, more like thousands of pounds. Anyway, chap got sent down. Ford Open Prison, you know. Well believe it or not the chap …'

At that point, two more of the registrars left Sister's office to answer their bleeps.

MacLeod whispered to Bonehead,

'You know what the registrars are up to, don't you, Bonehead? The bastards are bored, aren't they? They're tired of the round and the Muffin chatter. So when one of them got lucky and was bleeped out of the office, he's taken the opportunity of bleeping the others out of the round and rescuing them. They've probably pissed off to the mess and are out there giggling over a game of pool.'

'Spect so, don't blame the bastards.'

At that point, MacLeod's own bleep went off. The consultants turned and looked quizzically at him, their looks commenting on the vulgarity of housemen, generally, and on the temerity of MacLeod for interrupting their conversation, specifically.

'Would you mind if I answered my bleep, Sir?'

'If you really must, MacLeod. Mind you, only this once and it had better be important. If I recall correctly, the last time that wretched bleep of yours went off, it was your stockbroker.'

MacLeod glanced towards the door and to his amazement saw the office door push open and the registrars shuffle back in to Sister's office.

'Goodness me,' he thought, 'they weren't playing pool after all.'

MacLeod stood at Sister's desk and dialled the number that had registered on his bleep. The phone was answered almost immediately.

'Dr MacLeod, is that you? It's Stephanie Miller speaking. Dr MacLeod, you're the chairman of the Doctors' Mess aren't you?'

'Who am I speaking to, please?'

'Stephanie Miller. I am the hospital's deputy chief executive.'

'Ah.'

MacLeod felt a momentary surge of panic and stroked back his hair with an anxious movement of his left hand. Sensing an evolving drama, the consultants stopped chatting and watched MacLeod with interest. Wilson gawped at MacLeod, came to attention and put his tea on Sister's desk, an unheard-of impropriety.

'Dr MacLeod, you are chairman of the Doctors' Mess?'

'Ah yes, I am. They couldn't find anyone else to do the job you see.'

'Well never mind that. I am very glad that I am speaking to the right man. Now look here, was there a party in the Mess last night?'

'A party?' MacLeod gulped. 'No. Why do you ask?'

There was silence in Sister's office and the faces of the consultants, nurses and junior doctors focused with a curious intensity on MacLeod and his conversation.

'Dr MacLeod, I do have here a most peculiar situation, do you see? I am speaking to you on behalf of my colleagues. They're here with me now. Are you sure there wasn't a party in the hospital last night?'

'Yes, I'm sure there wasn't.'

'May I continue, Dr MacLeod?'

'Of course.'

'Dr MacLeod, have you had the slightest intimation that there has been a disturbance in the Management Offices? Dr MacLeod? Have you heard that all of our desks have been removed from our offices?'

'No. I didn't know ... that ...'

MacLeod had great difficulty in restraining his laughter and clasped the mouthpiece of the phone tightly hoping to muffle all sounds.

'Well, they have all been removed. And what's more, Dr MacLeod, the beds have been replaced with desks. We're most ...'

MacLeod could no longer control himself and guffawed. An explosion of laughter cascaded around the room and billowed from the walls. The consultant rose from their chairs and stared at him.

'... most concerned. And, do you know the perpetrators have jolly well gone and arranged our computers and phones and photographs on the beds? Nothing has been lost, nothing has been stolen. It's bizarre in the extreme. Can you imagine how puzzling this is to us all in Hospital Management?'

MacLeod, writhing with silent laughter, laughter that was painful, caught Wilson's eye and oblivious to the gawping of Sister and the senior medical staff, the pair hugged, slapped each other on the back, and fell on the floor, the muffled phone still clasped in MacLeod's hand.

MacLeod managed to stop laughing for the briefest moment to reiterate from the floor of Sister's office that there hadn't been a doctor's party in the hospital the previous night. As MacLeod, hugging Wilson, looked up from the floor, he saw between bouts of laughter, both of the consultants standing over him with puzzled expressions on their faces. The consultants loomed over the pair as they rolled on the floor, rattling with laughter.

'MacLeod! Wilson! What on earth is going on here?'

'Sorry, Sir. I'll tell you in a moment, Sir. Sorry.'

MacLeod struggled to his feet and removed his hand from the phone. Wilson remained on the floor convulsed with laughter. The consultants backed away and, returning to their seats, stared at MacLeod with puzzlement. The registrars gawped and the nurses paid them no attention at all but conferred about rotas and ward schedules.

'So, you were saying, Mrs Miller, that nothing has been stolen? That's very good news.'

'Yes, but Dr MacLeod, that's not the point is it? Nothing may have been stolen but criminals have broken into our rooms and removed our desks. There is a clear security risk here. What are we to do? But you say, Dr MacLeod that there wasn't any party, no unseemly behaviour last night. If you're sure about that, then I suppose it can't have been the doctors. It must have been the medical students then?'

'I doubt it was the medical students. It certainly doesn't sound like it could possibly have been the medical students.'

'Ah, so you do think then that it was the doctors?'

MacLeod straightened his jacket and hunched his shoulders.

'Yes, it sounds to me like it was the doctors. Leave it to me, Mrs Miller. I will make enquiries immediately and try to find the culprits. I'll get back to you as soon as I possibly can. I'll make it a priority. I'll call you back shortly.'

MacLeod put down the phone. Meanwhile, Wilson had got up from the floor and still roaring with laughter, hugged MacLeod, and then threw him up in the air and caught him. MacLeod detached himself from Wilson's embrace and looked around at the incredulous stares of the doctors and nurses.

'I think you owe us an explanation,' said Mr Cowie, crossing and then uncrossing his legs. 'Now, MacLeod, as you will see, I am sitting comfortably, and as I am sitting comfortably, you, MacLeod, may begin. Come, let's hear it. Speak up.'

MacLeod described what had happened to an awed audience.

Mr Cowie beamed at MacLeod, and commented wryly,

'Quite the most marvellous thing since Mr D R Davies's Ford Anglia was taken up one night in the lift to the operating theatres and driven into the centre of Operating Suite One.'

And the slightly complacent smile on Mr Cowie's face as he recounted the story of the Anglia, mirrored by the expression on Mr Bailey's face, left Doctors MacLeod and Wilson in no doubt as to who had been involved in that particular jape all those years ago.

Chapter 7
The Driving Offence

MacLeod was driving to work. It was 8.30 am on a Monday morning and he was due on duty in Cambridge at 9 am. He'd spent the weekend off duty in North London where he'd enjoyed himself. It had been a weekend of old friends, parties and sleep, which was in considerable contrast with life at the hospital which consisted of new friends, parties and no sleep.

MacLeod was in good time for work. He had to be punctual because he was on call that day. 'On call' meant that he was 'on take' in Casualty and was responsible for holding the cardiac arrest bleep. For MacLeod, apart from arrest bleep dramas, life on take in Cambridge was generally uneventful as there were very few admissions.

The traffic between North London and Cambridge hadn't been too bad and, driving against the riptide of the commuter rush, MacLeod had the pleasure of contrasting the ease of his journey into Cambridgeshire with the view of cars queuing on their way into town. It wasn't exactly schadenfreude but it was a near enough feeling that MacLeod embraced as he contemplated the lines of cars stacked neatly up against traffic lights and roundabouts. In his Mini, the heater rattled and clouds of damp air tainted with engine oil and exhaust gases gusted around the car. Heating the Mini was a balance of risks. The choice was between frostbite or death by carbon monoxide poisoning. When MacLeod felt close to suffocation he turned the heating off. When he could no longer feel his toes, the heater went back on. The Mini was a magnificent

J. Waxman, *MacLeod's Introduction to Medicine*,
DOI 10.1007/978-1-4471-4522-6_7,
© Springer-Verlag London 2014

antique. Rust spots spattered the paintwork and an enamel AA badge decorated the radiator grill.

The countryside passed by pleasantly, the new green of the trees beautiful in the spring's bright sunshine. The radio was on and the *Today* programme was in full flow. Some poor cabinet minister was being exquisitely tortured by an interviewer, who completely unreasonably was insisting that he had a straightforward answer to a simple question, an answer that was impossible to give if he wanted to maintain the prime minister's confidence and remain in office. MacLeod and four million listeners had no sympathy at all for the minister's pain. The interviewer ratcheted up the thumbscrews and the minister squealed ...

'If you could give me just a moment, I could answer your question ...'

'Certainly, Minister ...'

But the answer related to a policy triumph in another unrelated area and was quite irrelevant to the interviewer's question which was not surprisingly repeated. MacLeod chuckled as the minister squirmed.

The Mini passed on through Hertfordshire's villages, through narrow roads designed for carthorses but not forty ton trucks, where the windows and walls of roadside houses were spattered with road kill, mud and grime. The Mini rattled over rumble strips, slowing at crossings, obeying the dire warnings that pedestrians, old people, deer, elephants, chickens and children were about to cross the road. 'Beware' and MacLeod braced himself, ready for the unshackled triceratops that was about to jump into his path.

In the bare countryside again, gulls wheeled over naked fields, calling, cackling, while a red tractor pulled a plough, earth spilling up and over its blades. In the cities and towns of MacLeod's life, there were pavements and houses, shops and crowds. Every time that he drove out of London, he faced anew the revelation that England was not entirely urban and that there was a pastoral life unnoticed by urbanites.

Ten minutes passed and the interviewer's incisions without anaesthetic on the cabinet minister ceased. It was time for the

sports roundup and the programme continued with the
chirpy news of yet another glorious England Test defeat, and
onwards and upwards to a fabulous quarter-final tennis disaster. As the commentator joked with the defeated stars,
MacLeod, looking in his rear-view mirror, noticed a car
creeping closer and closer to his rear bumper. The proximity
of the car agitated him. It was too close, and disturbed the
even tenor of his journey to Cambridge. MacLeod accelerated a little to keep a safe distance between his Mini and the
car on his tail. The road was single lane, narrowed by an
arcade of trees. MacLeod lowered his window and shouted,

'Overtake, you bastard!' and, in response, a squadron of
pigeons tumbled from the trees above.

But MacLeod's pursuer couldn't overtake; there was just
no room on the road for two cars abreast of each other. The
car edged closer.

'Crikey,' thought MacLeod, 'he's in a hurry.' And he accelerated to get away.

But MacLeod was still not going fast enough for the driver
of the Ford Mondeo who kept close to the Mini's back bumper, too close, in MacLeod's view, for safety. MacLeod put his
foot down further on the Mini's throttle. The speedometer
registered 45 mph, quite fast enough in MacLeod's view for a
Monday morning drive in the country. But the man on his tail
seemed dissatisfied with progress and made no concession to
MacLeod's increased speed. He was still there hanging on to
the Mini's bumper, too close for comfort.

'What an idiot,' thought MacLeod, 'I'm not going any
faster. He can nob off.'

The Mondeo edged closer and, with a sigh, MacLeod
pressed down on the accelerator pedal and the Mini edged
faster. The car was going at 50 mph which was almost at the
antique's limit. MacLeod had travelled at 60 mph, once, but
that was when the car was a puppy and when MacLeod had
been trying to terrify his mother into increasing his medical
school allowance. As might have been predicted, his attempt
at blackmail had failed badly and his allowance had been
stopped.

The cavalcade of two cars sped into yet another Hertfordshire village and despite his efforts to shake off the Ford, the car was still glued to the Mini's bumper.

'What's the guy on?' MacLeod growled to himself, and for answer came there silence.

But still the car behind him was forcing MacLeod to go faster and faster, driving too close, pushing him to the car's limit. There was no place in the narrow country lanes for the Mondeo to pass and so MacLeod responded to the maniac by driving a little faster and then a lot faster.

'This is ridiculous! I don't want to go faster.'

And MacLeod slowed to a sedate 45 mph which seemed to get the driver behind him even more irritated. By now he'd been pursuing MacLeod for at least ten minutes and at every point in the pursuit there had been no opportunity for him to pass. MacLeod wound the window down and cool country air swept into the interior. He rested his elbow on the sill and tried to relax but the guy behind him wouldn't let him drive at a comfortable speed.

'This is absurd!'

And MacLeod stabbed at the accelerator pedal, attempting to get away from the Mondeo's embrace. But the attempt was useless and the driver of the Mondeo stuck close matching MacLeod's speed with his speed. It was a duet for idiots, through bends and over zebra crossings, a duet for fools suddenly punctuated by the shrieking lunacy of a siren.

'The police!' MacLeod announced to the *Today* programme. 'About time too! They'll sort him out. The police are after the bugger.'

MacLeod looked smugly into his rear-view mirror, expecting to see a troop of police cars ringed around the Mondeo. But there were none. He couldn't see a single patrol car nudging the speeding driver to the curb. However, what MacLeod *could* see when he looked in the mirror was a blue light on the roof of the Mondeo and a gesticulating Mondeo driver urging MacLeod to pull over to the side of the road. So MacLeod did as he was bid, but it was an indignant MacLeod who slowed down, a MacLeod roused to incandescence by the injustice of his situation. MacLeod was furious and he roared,

'I'm innocent. The bugger pushed me into speeding. I was just trying to avoid being rammed. It's an outrage! What a bastard!' But to nobody's surprise there was no reply from the *Today* program.

MacLeod and his Mini turned in to the side of the road. The Mondeo pulled up behind the Mini and a uniformed policeman got out of the car. The officer slammed the car door shut, put his helmet on and adjusted its tilt. Backlit in stroboscopic blue, the policeman strolled with some considerable deliberation towards MacLeod. The menace of his approach reminded MacLeod of a lion creeping up on an iguana.

The policeman stood by the passenger door of the Mini, and unleashed a notebook and a biro from his jacket pocket. He flicked open the book and, licking his thumb, turned to a fresh charge sheet.

Then he bent to look through the window at MacLeod, and MacLeod, staring at the policeman, saw an open-mouthed image of himself reflected in the eyes of the law. The policeman straightened up, and slowly, with heavy and deliberate footsteps, walked to the front of the car to take down the Mini's registration number. MacLeod got out of the car and stepped on to the pavement. He watched the policeman writing in a laboured fashion, the heavily impressed biro marking the dimensions of MacLeod's Hell-toasted misdemeanours. The policeman completed the entry in his notebook and looked up at MacLeod.

'I must advise you, Sir, that you have committed an offence and that anything that you might choose to say will be taken down and used in evidence against you ...'

The weight of the pause in the policeman's statement was so heavy it seemed to MacLeod to exceed the known weight of the universe.

'The bastard!' he thought, 'The *evil black-hearted* bastard. How could he do that to me? It was bloody well him that was speeding, not me. *He* made me go faster, the swine. Blasted police! There I was just tootling along minding my own business until he came along behind me and pushed me to go faster. And because he seemed to want to get past me and there was no bloody room to pass, I went faster. It was his blasted fault – not mine!'

The policeman, unaware of the tenor of MacLeod's thoughts continued to make notes. Clouds of anger coalesced in MacLeod's heart and bubbled up into a boiling storm of bilious black rage.

'Anything I might choose to say? I bloody well *do* have something to say ...'

And MacLeod with admirable presence of mind continued,

'I was travelling to Addenbrooke's Hospital in Cambridge where I have to be on duty at 9 o'clock, and hold the cardiac arrest bleep ...

MacLeod pointedly tugged at his coat sleeve and looked down at his watch.

'...and you have made me late.'

The policeman stopped writing, looked up from his note-pad and gawped at MacLeod, mouth wider than the Blue Nile.

'Please write that down, officer. And don't forget the last bit. I'll repeat it for you just in case. And you have made me late. Got that have you? And you have made me late.'

The policeman gulped and, tipping his helmet back, scratched his head.

'May I see your driving licence, Sir?' And after checking the details, gave it back to him. 'You may complete your journey, Sir.'

MacLeod returned to his seat shaking with indignation, vibrating with a fury made incandescent by the trap into which he'd been tipped by the policeman's driving.

'So bloody unfair ...' he thought, as he completed the final fifteen miles of his journey to Cambridge. But his mood calmed as the miles faded, and he rolled into the hospital car park only a few minutes late for handover.

It was a quiet Monday in Casualty with its usual roll call of drug overdoses, alcohol excesses and sexually transmitted diseases, all problems for which the nurses and doctors on duty for the day needed treatment before they could be reasonably expected to deal with the tidal wave of patients who swamped the waiting area. It was a relaxing day, otherwise, and MacLeod was able to go from Casualty to carry out a ward round of the thin-skinned, stick-boned mass of anorexic patients whom the professor was treating with infusions of a particular jungle juice. There was no logical basis for the infusions that any medical person apart from the bonkers professor could ascertain. But who on this earth would go against the views of a distinguished Cambridge professor?

The professor's clinical standards were generally bizarre. He treated heart failure with laxatives and respiratory complaints with antidepressants. Patients with any serious illness who came under his care were subject to the oddest experimentation. As a result, the professor's success rate was low, and few were cured by his approach to medicine. Word of the professor's eccentricities got out, and it was whispered in the community that he was to be avoided at all costs, because his touch was the kiss of death. And the consequence was that, after a few years of professorial life at Addenbrooke's, no GP referred any patients to the professor for review in outpatient clinics.

The professor's only chance for new patient referral came when he was on emergency take. The emergency take rota was very rigidly structured at Addenbrooke's. Every consultant had his regular day on call. The professor's day on take was Monday, and counterintuitively, although Monday take started at 9 am on Monday, it finished on Tuesday at 9 am. Knowing of the madness of the professor of medicine, the local GPs avoided referring patients to Casualty on Mondays. The GPs' patients were managed at home for as long as possible with the hope that prayer and the judicious application of antibiotics, poultices and diuretics would tide them over to the period when a rational hospital consultant with conventional thought processes would be in charge of casualty admissions. All the more mobile and sentient patients either opted for a bus trip to a neighbouring hospital for treatment or waited for the clock to hit 9 am on Tuesday before dialling 999.

In a way, MacLeod rather enjoyed his post as house officer to the professor, its quietness and absence of Casualty GP referrals was a beautiful interlude of tranquillity compared with the roaring pace of his previous post.

MacLeod's Monday passed uneventfully; the two very ill patients who couldn't possibly have put off admission because of the seriousness of their conditions and lack of mobility had been dealt with immaculately. Because there had been no other work to do, these two patients had been blessed by the quality of attention that the Queen or her consort might have received had they chanced to have been brought into Casualty. Investigations were ordered immediately, drips set up within moments and referrals to other services organised within panache and aplomb.

On her way out of Casualty on a lumbering trolley taking her to X-ray, half of Macleod's admissions had cranked herself up on an elbow and said,

'It's wonderful, the NHS. Couldn't have been better if I'd gone private, dear.' And MacLeod had nodded his agreement.

So, for MacLeod, the day's take had been a peaceful arrangement of leisurely diagnoses and academic discourse with his ribald colleagues, who were jealous of MacLeod's gift of a peaceful take day. His colleagues rushed from one medical emergency to another whilst MacLeod had another coffee, scratched himself leisurely and got on with reading both *Grazia* and *Hello* magazines in great detail. MacLeod hoped that the material covered in these learned journals would help him pass his membership to the Royal College of Physicians, but this unfortunately was not very likely.

The only blip in the pleasant tenor of MacLeod's beautiful days on the wards at Addenbrooke's had a human form. That human form was embodied in the wart-enamelled person of a certain ward sister. Sister Crippen was rather short. Her uniform was unnaturally crisp, stiffened by pure thoughts and the ill wishes of past housemen. She was a straight-sided woman with a paranoid squint and a monstrous moustache. MacLeod wondered if the moustache had been dyed for gravitas. Sister Crippen's hands were reddened by obsessive washing and her dandruff-flecked hair was pulled tight from her skull by the ferocious grip of a hair clip with a sidereal sparkle. None of her physical irregularities were her fault, of course, but they were a reflection of the ugliness of Sister Crippen's miserable mind.

Sister Crippen was deeply religious, religious in an evangelical way that strove for the salvation of her staff nurses' souls, a process that was regularly thwarted by the efforts of MacLeod to find his own salvation through those very same souls. Sister Crippen and MacLeod were engaged in an essential struggle for the souls of the staff nurses – she likened his efforts to those of the Devil whilst he likened her efforts to those of an uglier, more warty version of the same sort of thing. MacLeod's aims were pure, his mind focusing on the political and intellectual development of those angels in female form. It was his ambition to help them realise their full potential, even if meant taking them to the pub to do so. As a result of this and many other of MacLeod's selfless activities, Sister Crippen had come unfairly to the view that MacLeod was a simulacrum of a human whose external form clothed a cesspool of black pus and vomit and a heart on loan from Loch Ness.

Monday take night had been a night of unbroken sleep for MacLeod. Casualty had not called and the wards had been peaceful. It was ever thus working for the professor and such a contrast with the lives on take of his colleagues, where the bustle of disease in all its malevolence filled all their weary hours.

MacLeod got up early to make ready for the post-take ward round. He dressed, shaved, ate breakfast and then rushed to the ward to write up the notes and check results. MacLeod stood stooped over the notes trolley frantically updating his patients' records. There was quiet on the wards, the patients tidied into their beds in expectation of the professor's rounds. The ward clock raced to 9 am. The ward swing doors pushed open and the professor, ignoring MacLeod, strode into the ward, knocked on the door of Sister's office and walked in, closing the door behind him.

Over the months of his house job, MacLeod had observed the professor's routine to be entirely predictable. The professor consistently arrived on the wards at the stroke of 9 am keen to go round the admissions, concerned that he carried out his duties meticulously. It was MacLeod's role to be on the wards when he arrived, to be part of the greeting party of doctors and nurses. The professor always wore grey, his single-breasted suit borrowed from a bank clerk, although his college tie was likely to be his own. The professor's hair was parted on the right and slicked back with a good dose of pomade; his shoes gleamed and his footsteps had the crisp retort of shattering ice.

The door to Sister's office swung open, and the professor, followed by a line of senior doctors and nurses, strode out into the ward and made their his way to MacLeod and the notes trolley. MacLeod straightened up to greet the professor and his jolly entourage.

'Hello, Prof!' was greeted by the curtest of nods.

The doctors and nurses clustered together around the notes trolley at the side of the tiny doctor's desk in the centre of the ward. The professor pulled out the medical folder of the first of his three in-patients. He was obsessive in his review of the patients' records. Stooped over the trolley, he rustled through the clerking notes and checked every single blood result, peering at the pages of medical records. As he flicked through sheaves of results, the professor seemed lost in his thoughts, rarely commenting on a patient's management, only concerned that processes had been followed, and results noted and dealt with.

The professor's ward rounds were formal and required that MacLeod should present each patient to the professor. He was not allowed to make his presentations with reference to the patients' records – these were for the professor's inspection. Each folder was opened in turn and spread out on the trolley. The professor thumbed through the notes and sought out MacLeod's clerking. As MacLeod gave the patient's history, the professor's index finger traced MacLeod's words on the page, his finger following his presentation line by line.

The day seemed strange and oppressive to MacLeod. The ward seemed tense. As MacLeod presented his first case to the professor, it felt as though the silence of the ward was following him and as if the eyes of the nearly dead and the merely sick were focused on him, as if pestilence and plague, sickness and malaise were hanging on his every word.

As the professor scanned the patients' notes, the senior registrar, the two registrars, sister and two staff nurses stood to attention, waiting on his comments, attentive and professional. MacLeod was somehow not of that group. He was a stranger on the outside of the circle of doctors and nurses, a stranger observing Medicine's manners.

MacLeod was amused to note that the posture of the senior registrar mirrored that of the professor, the senior registrar bent down over the notes trolley when the professor bent and straightened up when the professor stood up. The senior registrar glared at the registrars when the professor glared. His lips followed the professor's questioning of the juniors, forming silent words that echoed his consultant's words. The senior registrar smiled at the ward sister when the professor smiled at the frightful harridan, but unlike the professor's smiles, his smiles were not returned by her. Sister Crippen stood stock still, her eyes only on the professor, the curl of her lips flickering only for the professor, waiting for his comments, a handmaiden for his needs.

MacLeod didn't attempt any exchange of even the most superficial of courtesies with Sister Crippen. It was a waste of his time. She didn't speak to him, unless forced by the most extraordinary circumstance. She didn't look at him, except by accident. When MacLeod spoke, her demeanour became a fortress state of crossed-arm rigidity. Sister Crippen made it obvious that she loathed and despised him, hated him with a febrile candour, abhorred him with a rancid fervour. Sister Crippen's feelings for MacLeod boiled and bubbled, and from the volcano of her opprobrium, sour clouds of rumbling rancour erupted and spilled out onto the ward linoleum. Sister Crippen avoided any sight of him, was deaf to his voice and only breathed air that had avoided his lungs. In his presence, her moustache bristled and her squint expanded to fill her face.

But regardless of Sister Crippen's approbation, the ward round was going well. Two of the professor's patients had been presented by MacLeod and no fault had been found. The professor had listened to the cases, agreed with the diagnoses and had supported the need for the investigations ordered.

'Quite right!' he'd said and this was equivalent to anyone else's 'Well done!'.

At this, the senior registrar sniffed and Sister Crippen shuffled and glared. MacLeod went on to present one of the previous week's admissions, a poor old boy who'd been picked up unconscious on the street. The man had been found to have had a stroke and looked like he might never recover. MacLeod had phoned the man's GP and had managed to get from him a history of poorly controlled hypertension. On that basis, the stroke was considered likely to have been haemorrhagic, and unfortunately that diagnosis was correct.

'Good, good,' said the professor stroking his chin and smiling broadly.

The professor seemed pleased with the diagnosis, and MacLeod thought, 'How odd!'.

It was very strange to be delighted at misfortune of others, but it emerged that the reason that the professor was so thrilled was nothing to do with his pleasure at sharpness of MacLeod's clinical acumen. No, the professor was simply pleased that the correct investigations had been carried out in the correct order.

It was now 9.30 am, and MacLeod was ecstatic that things were going well. There had been no hiccough on the ward round and with the final patient presented, the group of doctors and nurses were getting ready for the long drift around the patients. It was almost time for the meet and greet section of the professor's regal procession from the throne room of his research laboratory to the bedsides of the sick. MacLeod knew that the professor enjoyed his rounds, liked the time spend standing over the sick, palpating this, listening to that, and all the while reminiscing, in his anecdotage about the famous clinicians who'd taught him as a student and junior doctor. And although he felt in his heart that he shouldn't,

MacLeod quite liked the stories, almost enjoyed the rambling relics of a time long since gone.

So, back to the patient and MacLeod continued his story of the poor old fellow with a stroke, the GP, the CT scan, the haemorrhage, the lack of recovery, the need to consider long-term social care, the wait for a possible secondary haemorrhage, which might be the best outcome all things considered. But it was the professor's view that in the context of a stroke, it was early days. He felt that the patient shouldn't be written off as there might be neurological recovery even though the present situation looked dire.

And it was just at that point that MacLeod's bleep went off. The bleep punctuated the professor monologue on the possibility of late recovery from major stroke, but the professor carried on regardless, ignoring the bleep's interruption. MacLeod seized the opportunity to take a stealthy glance at his bleep's display and saw that he had an outside call. In MacLeod's view, outside calls were the only reason to have a bleep, allowing the junior doctor additional contact beyond mobile phones with the outside world.

'I'll take that for you, Dr MacLeod.'

MacLeod was startled by the offer. It was Sister Crippen, who'd skipped around the notes trolley and was standing in front of him, hand outstretched to take the bleep from him and answer his call.

'How extraordinary!' he thought. 'She never does that! Answer my bleep! Crikey! She's more likely to throw a bedpan at me than answer my bleep.'

'Thank you, Sister.'

Trying to suppress a look of amazement at this unusual generosity, MacLeod handed Sister Crippen his bleep. She took it from him, looked at the display and went to the ward office to take the call, stalking away from the ward round, the thump of her heels on the ward floor reverberating through the entire structure of the hospital, rattling the drip stands, shaking the beds and rocking the notes trolley.

The professor's attempts to educate his juniors continued, with a history of neurosurgical intervention in haemorrhagic stroke. It seemed that the professor had personally known all the great clinicians who had made any sort of contribution to the subject. MacLeod looked around at his colleagues and noted the glazed look in their eyes as they daydreamed of anything, of anything other than the history of surgical interventions in haemorrhagic stroke.

The thump of Sister Crippen's footsteps grew closer, and she re-joined the little group of doctors and nurses around the trolley. A smile played at the edges of her lips. MacLeod was curious to know the cause of this smile. He had not seen her smile before. MacLeod stared at Sister Crippen with puzzlement. And then Sister Crippen coughed violently. One of the junior registrars looked up at her, his attention caught by her coughing. She coughed again more loudly, and the rest of the group looked up and stared at her, apart from the professor, who was lost in his exposition of the causes, treatment and outlook of haemorrhagic stroke.

'**Ahemmmmmmm!**' she spluttered.

Her coughing fit caught the attention of everyone from the professor to the ward clerk. The ward cleaner stopped mopping and the X-ray porter ceased pushing a wheelchair through the ward and looked at Sister Crippen. Every patient in every bed was transfixed. What was the matter with Sister Crippen? The coughing continued, until that point when even the professor stopped talking.

'Are you all right, Sister?' the professor asked solicitously. 'Would you like a glass of water?'

The ward was hushed; all attention was concentrated on Sister Crippen. Silence reigned and, apart from the coughing, there was no other noise. And then, attention garnered, the coughing suddenly stopped. An unpleasant gleam appeared in Sister Crippen's eyes. A complacent smirk crept over her face. Her squint became exaggerated. Sister Crippen's moustache bristled. The professor looked anxiously at Sister Crippen and the registrars stared.

The eyes of all upon her, Sister Crippen turned dramatically to MacLeod and in the loudest of voices boomed,

'**Dr MacLeod, It's the police. They want to speak to you.**'

Sister Crippen smirked with the deepest satisfaction and the assembled team of doctors and nurses gawped at MacLeod.

It was as if Sister Crippen had been waiting for that call from the moment two months ago when MacLeod had set foot on her ward. With that call, which she had the foresight and intuition to take, she had been given the evidence that confirmed her view that MacLeod was deeply bad. Sister Crippen had always known in her heart that MacLeod was evil. She contemplated the options ...

'Is he a serial killer? Is he a thief? A murderer? Had he committed unspeakable crimes? Whatever his villainy, and he's surely a criminal, here's evidence that he's up to no good, that he's been responsible for the worst of crimes against humanity.'

And here, with this phone call, was the vindication that Sister Crippen had been waiting for. This call from the Baldock Police Station desk sergeant was the call that she had known would come, some time, some day. And that time was now – today was a good day for Sister Crippen. She had known all along that MacLeod was evil. And was satisfied now she was right.

Sister Crippen shuffled the sweet mass of satisfaction around in her mind and smirked. She felt very good. She felt very good indeed. Sister Crippen savoured victory; Sister Crippen sucked on righteousness, and victory and righteousness tasted like parma violets.

The doctors and nurses stared at MacLeod, and the patients stared at MacLeod.

'Goodness!' they thought.

'What has he done?' They were shocked. They felt anxious.

'The police! The police calling the hospital! What on Earth has he been up to? What has he done! Bad boy! The police?'

'Must be serious! Gracious! And goodness me, he's touched me. That doctor, he's had his hands on my bits.'

But there was no element of shock in Sister Crippen's mind. She had always known her man. She had known him from the start, known that MacLeod was bad.

'Those poor girls that he's tempted! Well, don't say that I didn't warn them right from the start. I told them he was a villain. And now here's that call from the police. They've caught up with him at last. He's a criminal. They'll come to get him shortly, come and take him into custody. He'll be in prison for years.'

Sister Crippen's smile extended beyond her face. It felt good to her that justice was at last on its way. It was such a relief to her that Her Majesty's prison's cells would be cosseting MacLeod in their unforgiving depths.

Sister Crippen decided that she would repeat her words now that she had everyone's full attention.

'The police, Dr MacLeod, the police,' she echoed.

'They're on the phone. You're *wanted*, you know.'

And the happiest of smiles spread joyously across her miserable face. Sister Crippen chuckled happily, her thoughts dallying with images of MacLeod in the dock, MacLeod in prison, MacLeod hanging by the neck …

'You better take the call, Dr MacLeod,' spluttered the professor.

MacLeod was puzzled, MacLeod was concerned, MacLeod was just a little bit worried about the unknown crime with which he was about to be confronted.

MacLeod walked to Sister's office, the eyes of all of the patients, doctors and nurses following his progress. He opened the office door and took up the receiver from where it lay on Sister's desk, amidst copies of ward nursing rotas and theatre lists.

'Hello? This is MacLeod speaking.'

'Sergeant Crabbe here. Baldock Police.'

'How can I help you, Sergeant?'

'Ah, Dr MacLeod! Good to speak to you, Sir. Just checking …'

'Checking what, Sergeant?'

'Well, Doctor, one of my officers was on traffic duty on Monday and he booked you for speeding … and your statement was rather unusual. So I thought that I'd better check that you were a bona fide doctor …'

'I see, Sergeant. Well, I can confirm that I am who I say I am.'

'Thank you, Dr MacLeod. Having called the hospital, checked with the switchboard and with your ward sister and yourself, I think then we can conclude that you are, indeed, a doctor and that you did in fact have a legitimate reason to be travelling rather faster than you should have been ...'

MacLeod held his breath at this point in the conversation.

'... and furthermore I am able to say that, in view of the circumstances and the nature of your statement, I am rather inclined to let the matter drop. We will not be pressing charges.'

'Thank you, Officer.'

'Goodbye, Doctor. And hopefully you won't be speeding again, will you, Doctor?'

'Certainly not, Sergeant.'

The phone line cut. MacLeod scratched his head and, with a grin, silently whooped to himself:

'Victory! I beat the bugger. It's a triumph of good over evil!'

MacLeod put down the receiver and returned to join the ward round where he found the doctors and nurses waiting for him. Their eyes were upon him as he closed the door of Sister's office and walked nonchalantly towards them.

'Well, MacLeod?' the professor asked.

'Yes, thank you, Professor. All very well indeed, as I'm sure Sister will be delighted to hear.'

But the look on Sister Crippen's face was more than a million miles from delight, as she contemplated the grin on MacLeod's face while he continued with the professor's ward round and moved on to assess the next patient.

Chapter 8
The Joys of Postgraduate Research

The years had gone by and as pen recorders had been edged out by more sophisticated means of measurement, MacLeod was hopeful that, with the passage of time, his research career might meet with a greater chance of success. MacLeod's period in postgraduate research followed on from his house jobs, senior house jobs and registrar training – time well spent in the company of loose women, time well spent in bars and snooker halls with inappropriate companions. MacLeod had been blessed by this traditional postgraduate education and had been fortunate in his training to amass volumes of information on the ways of all flesh. And so, armed with his years as a junior and senior junior doctor, MacLeod felt that it was time to spill his seed on the soil of research and hope that he remained fertile despite any past indiscretions.

MacLeod found employment at St Bartholomew's Hospital in the City of London. The hospital had been founded in the Middle Ages and its buildings carried the weight of the centuries with grace. MacLeod enjoyed walking though Bart's ancient arched Henry VIII gateway and into the courtyard bordered by stone-clad ward blocks of varying vintage. In the courtyard, a tall fountain trickled onto a tarry pool where fat goldfish cruised in its depths. Ancient plane trees surrounded the fountain and at dusk, dense legions of starlings swept screeching into the square and, landing in the high planes, made their play for the night.

J. Waxman, *MacLeod's Introduction to Medicine*,
DOI 10.1007/978-1-4471-4522-6_8,
© Springer-Verlag London 2014

In the daytime, the square was a thoroughfare for the sick, a meeting place for doctors and nurses, a car park for the consultants, a rendezvous for visitors. Medical students monopolised benches, porters smoked behind bicycle sheds and regular drug deals were hatched by Rastafarians from Hackney and other distant climes.

MacLeod found himself to be the only candidate interviewed for his research post. The odds for employment were favourable, he thought – or if they found him out, unfavourable. But after some desultory questioning, the interview committee chairman nodded encouragingly at MacLeod, thanked him for applying for the position and asked his colleagues on the interview panel if they had any questions for their candidate. There were no further questions, apart from,

'When can you start?'

And that seemed to be it.

MacLeod was employed to carry out research into fertility in Hodgkin's disease, which mainly affects young people and which until the mid-1960s had been fatal. Chemotherapy had been developed in the'60s and cured most patients. However treatment was associated with side-effects, the most significant of which was infertility. The drugs used in the treatment programme were directly toxic to the testes and ovaries, destroying sperm and ova. MacLeod's research job was to catalogue the effects of the chemotherapy, establishing whether the sterilising effect was universal, whether or not there was recovery and whether there was a sex difference in the toxic effects of treatment.

Before being set loose on patients, MacLeod was asked by the professor of oncology to arrange to see the professor of endocrinology at Barts, as he would be working closely with colleagues in the endocrinology department. Apparently, the previous occupant of MacLeod's research post had bad manners, and her behaviour had alienated the oncology and endocrinology departments. The purpose of MacLeod's interview was to see whether he had sufficiently good manners to mend relationships. Accordingly, doing entirely as he was told, MacLeod made an appointment to meet the professor of endocrinology and some six weeks later sat in his office establishing relationships.

The office was small and lined with bookshelves that appeared stable, unlike Dr Williams' bookshelves. The office was dominated by a huge desk that, in contrast to Dr Williams' desk, was completely uncluttered. The professor was very tall, very tanned, and immaculately dressed. Because of the bookshelves, the lack of clutter and, most critically, the professor's dress sense, MacLeod felt that he might expect more effective research supervision this time around. The professor leaned forward to look at MacLeod, his chin resting on his fist, his elbow resting on his thigh, legs crossed and locked around each other in a complex curl. MacLeod perched on the edge of a chair that had been set far too close to the professor's chair. Their knees touched. The professor stared at MacLeod with shockingly bright blue eyes. MacLeod felt uncomfortable, felt as though he was being scanned and found wanting, felt as though he was being examined with what almost seemed to be a sexual interest.

'Are you sensitive?' asked the professor of endocrinology, opening up the conversation, and his blue-eyed stare pierced right into MacLeod's soul and made him squirm. MacLeod was not convinced that the links that the professor of endocrinology intended to establish with him were of the nature entirely intended by the professor of oncology when he had encouraged MacLeod to mend relationships.

But the professor's opening question required an answer.

'Possibly. I play the piano you know,' replied MacLeod, and then ground to a halt, quivering with the thought that he had said something completely inane in reply to the professor's question. And the professor, realising that MacLeod was not for him, covered for the innuendo in his question by continuing,

'... because you will be dealing with a subject that requires great sensitivity you know.'

MacLeod went back to the sixth-floor research office where he had been closeted with a dozen or so young research doctors. In their office, the young academics actively engaged in cutting-edge medical research. They spent their time wisely, drinking coffee industriously. In the lacunae of time between cups of coffee, the academics could be seen assiduously staring out of the grubby window onto a light well graced by pigeon shit and darkness.

In the course of a few months, MacLeod catalogued the effects of chemotherapy on fertility. He did so by measuring hormone levels in the women treated for Hodgkin's disease and found that they were mostly menopausal. He measured sperm counts in the men and discovered that the counts were very low. In moments spent with his coffee cups, he considered how far which patients would go at their doctor's request and was amazed that men were prepared to masturbate in order to produce the sperm samples needed to asses their fertility status. MacLeod found that around 80 % of men and women were sterilised by chemotherapy. They resumed their life afterwards but it was a sterile life. So, it wasn't the greatest of cures.

At lunch in the Doctors' Mess, sitting at a long refectory table, MacLeod leaned over his egg salad, the least poisonous of the day's options, and talked about his findings with his friends.

'Listen, guys, it's such a shame. The patients with HD, they're cured but sterile. Wish there was something that they could take to prevent the chemotherapy sterilising them. Anybody have any ideas? Is there something that we could do to help them?'

The attention of his peers waned, but MacLeod continued regardless,

'The thing is that chemotherapy is a non-specific poison. It affects rapidly dividing cells the most – that's how and why chemo works. Chemo doesn't distinguish between cancer cells and normal cells. It just kills all cells that are rapidly dividing, blood cells, cells in the gut and, of course, the sperm and ova. Now, if I had a drug that effectively could put the goolies to sleep during chemotherapy, and stop germ cells dividing, then maybe I could prevent the effects of chemotherapy on the gonads and stop the chemo from having a sterilising effect. There must be a way?'

MacLeod had become energised and waved his fork in the air to emphasise the importance of his subject. Bits of egg white flew off his fork and lodged unnoticed in his neighbour's hair.

His colleagues, wrapped up in last night's hangovers, dreaming of girls and nauseous from the effects of their ghastly curry lunch, were oblivious to MacLeod's chatter. No one paid him the slightest attention – except Roger. This was because Roger didn't have a hangover, had no need to dream of girls because there was the reality of a Mrs Roger, and hadn't been taken in by the sleazy enticements of a canteen curry because he had brought sandwiches to work. Roger was a languid Australian exported from the colonies by his hospital bosses to study endocrinology. Roger was quietly smart. He was tall and skinny with a flop of brown hair that fell from a right-sided parting to shield his eyes from the glare of the English sun. And those eyes had a curiously inquisitive way of staring straight out through that stream of hair. Yes, Roger was listening; Roger had a reputation for listening, listening quietly and then suddenly saying something of shocking and unexpected clarity.

MacLeod stopped mid-sentence wondering what on earth could be done to save the sperm. It was his mission to save the sperm. Other doctors may have had other missions on their minds but MacLeod was focused on Mission 'E', or to put it another way, 'E' Mission.

Roger wanted to know more about the patients with Hodgkin's disease.

'So, you say that chemo kills just the dividing cells, is that right?'

'Yes, that type of chemo, the type that you give to Hodgkin's patients, kills all rapidly dividing cells.'

'And you want to find a drug that will stop the cells in the gonads from dividing, a drug that will put the testes and ovaries in the freezer? Have I got that right?'

MacLeod nodded. Roger had, indeed, got that right.

'Well, MacLeod, there is such a drug. It was introduced to promote puberty. Unfortunately for the company that made it, the drug had no effect. Yes, one dose did transiently boost the hormones that control the gonads. But when the drug is given repeatedly, it has the opposite effect and switches off these hormones. So the drug has the potential to cause the testes and the ovaries to go into a resting state. Isn't that just the sort of drug that you want for your Hodgkin's patients? Give it a try? What's to lose? It's safe. It's entirely specific; give it a go?'

MacLeod was absorbed by Roger's arguments. Why not give it a go, indeed? In Medicine, in order to prove that a drug works, proof of effect has to be obtained in a placebo-controlled clinical trial where patients are randomly allocated to receive either the new experimental treatment or no treatment at all. In that way, there can be certainty of the effects of a new treatment.

MacLeod went away and buckled down to work. He got permission to use the drug for free from the drug company, and obtained ethical committee approval for the trial. After a while, the drug trial was up and running and MacLeod had time to sit and reflect. And this is what he thought …

'Now, MacLeod, you know you have got this drug. And you know that it can switch off the testes and ovaries. So, if it can do that in Hodgkin's disease, is the drug useful in any other condition?'

. And then the answer to his question beamed in from the ether, in a golden moment studded with huge sparkling diamonds.

'Of course, it's useful in other conditions – **prostate cancer**!'

At that time, the treatment of prostate cancer was by castration and treatment had been unchanged since the 1940s. MacLeod's view about this as a treatment for cancer was:

'Having to be castrated just because you have the misfortune to have cancer? That's a double whammy!'

So, MacLeod found Bill Hendry, a friendly urologist, and explained what he had in mind for patients with prostate cancer.

'By all means, MacLeod, why don't you have a go?'

So MacLeod tried out the drug on a prostate cancer patient and the drug worked. The prostate gland is at the base of the bladder and, because of its critical position, men with prostate cancer can have difficulty urinating. Prostate cancer spreads to bone and causes pain. From being in pain, his first patient became pain free, and from having difficulty peeing, he could piss like an elephant. There is a blood test that is raised in patients with prostate cancer and the level in MacLeod's first patient became that of a normal man.

Reading that first blood test result, MacLeod bubbled with exhilaration and then, within seconds, the bubble burst and he got on with his day job.

MacLeod's second trial patient ran a theatrical bookstall in a street market at St Giles' Circus in Covent Garden. In the run up to his diagnosis, he had trouble with his 'waterworks' but no pain. The waterworks trouble had brought him eventually to his doctor, who had sent him to Casualty to be sorted out. Casualty had booked him in to Mr Hendry's clinic and, finally, Mr Hendry had sent the man to MacLeod.

'You know what, Doctor?' the patient exclaimed telling MacLeod the story of his illness.

'Oooo, that pissing – you know, it got really bad, it did; very bad it was. When I was at the stall, well, I was running to the loo in the pub every ten minutes.

'No *seriously,* Doctor, it was *dreadful.* I needed to go every ten minutes. It was *awful.* And, of course, because I'm gay – you may not have realised that, Doctor – but that lot in the pub thought that I was going there cottaging, know what I mean? Oooo – did I get some looks from them in there? *Anyway,* I couldn't keep on leaving my stall, could I? You'll never guess what I did, Doctor? Of course, you won't guess, how could you guess?

'Well, Doctor, I went off to Zeitgeist, you know the S&M shop in Soho? I bought myself a long black rubber hose, you can imagine the sort, can't you, Doctor? Well, I strapped it on to my willy, cut off the end – of the hose, not my willy, silly – and taped the end of the hose into a hot-water bottle that I tucked into my sock.

'Well, Doctor, of course, that sorted everything out for a while – until I stopped peeing completely. Oh my God, was that terrifying! Still, they sorted me out in Casualty, bless them. They are so wonderful. And then you came along and made me better. Of course …' and his voice dropped to a whisper,

'I've lost all capacity, you know, but what good did all that malarkey do me, anyway? I tell you, Doctor, all it did was get me into trouble – in a way, having cancer's done me a favour. Done me a favour, it has.'

It was a eureka moment, MacLeod's big thing in his medical career, and a very big thing for patients who would no longer need to be castrated as treatment for prostate cancer. Although he did not know it at the time, other groups around the world were also looking at this drug as a treatment for prostate cancer and eventually the treatment became the standard.

It was MacLeod's duty as a research registrar to attend surgical ward rounds and sit in on surgical clinics. The primary purpose of this was to ensure that the management of the cancer patients by the surgeons was linked to care provided by the cancer doctors. The secondary purpose was to find and then recruit patients to participate in clinical trials. The high point of MacLeod's week was Mr Hendry's ward round. Rounds were conducted in a traditional fashion. The ward sister and the doctors on the firm would wait for the consultant's arrival, with scouts at various points in the hospital to alert them of his appearance on the premises.

The scouts were out not because of fear, but out of respect. The staff wanted to be 'ready and correct' for Mr Hendry, who was unaffected and modest, a quiet decent man who was admired and liked by his colleagues. He had the standing and appearance of a mid-nineteenth-century German cavalry officer, straight backed, clip haired, steely eyed. His surgical reputation was huge; he was called on to carry out operations that would be technically beyond any but the most talented of surgeons. Regardless of the esteem with which he was held, Mr Hendry remained a shy man. He was happiest in the operating theatre, preferring knife work to the fork work of surgical rounds and clinics.

Mr Hendry pushed tentatively through the swing doors and crossed the borders of the ward. He wore a brilliantly white coat and neat collar, with a pristine stethoscope the lonely content of crisp pockets. His shirt and tie were immaculate and his boots looked as though they had been polished by a regiment of riflemen. He came to a halt at the entrance to the ward, where he was greeted by Sister and a line of clean-faced doctors and nurses.

'Good morning, Sister.'

Sister Abernethy was old school. Fierce and proper, hair tied tightly back, stiff pinafore, starched wimple.

'Good morning, Mr Hendry. There are fifteen patients for you to see today.'

Mr Hendry remained at attention at the entrance to the ward awaiting Sister's permission to enter her domain, for hers were the drip stands, the staff nurses and the bedpans, her ward was her kingdom, its borders forever divine. The patients were waiting for Mr Hendry, waiting between neatly folded sheets. To an observer, it might have seemed that the patients' beds had been lined up by a giant with a parallelogram, so precisely were they arranged.

'Thank you, Sister. Shall we make a start?'

'Certainly, Mr Hendry. Would you like to go round?'

And the throng of doctors and nurses gathered around Mr Hendry sailed off into the ward, with Sister's permission granted, an anti-bacterial armada tilting against the evil navies of death and disease. Sister steered the flotilla to the first of Mr Hendry's patients. Every patient, no matter how sick, lay to attention in the centre of their narrow bed, beautiful sheets folded precisely over their chests, chin up, nose pointing to heaven.

MacLeod stood in the midst of the crowd clustered around the first patient's bed, and listened to the houseman give the patient's history. Mr Hendry, standing to attention, focused on the detail that interested him.

Sister was in harmony with Mr Hendry, a harmony that had developed from their years working together, and she knew exactly when Mr Hendry felt like moving on to the next patient. It almost needed no word to pass between them; they were an established couple assured of each other's intentions. But Mr Hendry, his mast of politeness unfurled, would invariably say, just as the ward round embarked to the next patient,

'Thank you, Sister.'

And Sister smiled beatifically at Mr Hendry, for he was her God. Mr Hendry, nodding at the patient, walked on to the next bed. The ward round cast its anchor at the second bed. The patient sat up and stared anxiously at the doctors and nurses, pyjama top unbuttoned, bed sheets pushed back. The houseman told the tale; the patient had been found to have bladder cancer, a nasty sort of bladder cancer, and was due to have his bladder removed. His ureters, the tubes that drain the kidneys into the bladder, would be diverted into an ileostomy. This is a pouch of small bowel that would be excised from its natural home and fashioned by Mr Hendry into an artificial bladder opening up onto the skin of the abdominal wall.

There was a significant risk of death from the procedure and the patient would need to be nursed in ITU after the operation. There were also major side-effects from surgery. In addition to needing a bag that would hold his urine, the patient would be impotent because the nerves that control erection would have been cut at operation. In MacLeod's view, these details needed to be explained to the patient, but they weren't discussed.

MacLeod observed that Mr Hendry's interest in the ward round had been pricked by the thought of a jolly good operation. Mr Hendry rubbed his hands together and then, holding them in front of him in the manner of a sixteenth-century saint painted by Raphael, interrupted the houseman's history, looked straight towards the frightened patient and declaimed from the bottom of his bed in a voice for the entire ward,

'Little bit of cancer, Mr Stevens. I will take it out. Any questions?'

Mr Hendry paused, waiting for questions, but from the patient's bed came no questions, only,

'No questions, Mr Hendry. Thank you, Mr Hendry. Thank you very much'

'Very good! Thank you, Sister. Next patient, please.'

A few days after the ward round, MacLeod sat in on clinic with another estimable surgeon, a famous urologist called Mr PR Little. 'PR Little' – quite the most wonderful name for a urologist! PR Little seemed austere, but beneath the veneer of inapproachability, there was warmth and sensitivity. His manner was clipped but humour pervaded all his terse utterances. He had been 'unwell' in his life,

'Snatched from the jaws of death, don't you know?'

He'd had TB as a child and had spent a couple of years in a sanatorium. Then, in his middle years, he'd had a massive heart attack on the wards. He'd collapsed in front of the juniors, nurses and patients in the course of his rounds, and had been resuscitated by the arrest team. In a scene of high drama, he'd been rushed off for emergency cardiac bypass surgery. A year after surgery, he'd had to have a kidney removed because of cancer. Mr Little's many dances with death had made him understand what it was like to be a patient, to know that wounds left scars. At his core, he was gentle and kind. But like every surgeon that MacLeod had come across, his conversational style, his communication skills, replete as they were with barked questions, did leave a little to be desired in the modern context of communicating with patients.

MacLeod sat with Mr Little in a small clinic room that seemed to date from the nineteenth century and appeared not to have changed since that time. Its contents were a feast of Victorian mahogany and peeling Victorian paint. MacLeod was keen to find patients with prostate cancer for trials of a new way of giving the drug that he'd found to be active in prostate cancer. When he'd initially tried out the new drug, it had been given either as a nasal snuff or as a daily injection. The drug continued to be effective, but the way that it was given was not convenient. Recognising this, research chemists had developed a new way of giving the drug once a month by a depot injection under the skin. In preclinical studies in animals, the release characteristics of the preparation were excellent and levels of the drug in blood were observed to be satisfactorily stable over the entire month.

'Great!' thought MacLeod, knowing that once-monthly injection would be far better than daily treatments.

MacLeod had looked forward to the time when the drug would become available for the first studies in men. That time had come and MacLeod was in the clinic with Mr Little, looking for patients with prostate cancer who would be willing to have the new formulation of the drug.

'Guinea pigs!' Mr Little barked. 'That's what you need, a couple of human guinea pigs. Shouldn't be a problem, old boy, there are.plenty of them snuffling about.'

Mr Little took a lace handkerchief from his sleeve and blew his nose very loudly.

'Next patient, Sister, and do hurry them in. I've lunch to get to, don't you know.'

The clinic door closed on a man in a tired suit with immaculate creases and brilliantly shined shoes who sat down in front of Mr Little's desk. Mr Little peered at the patient, whilst MacLeod scuffed through the patient's hospital records to discover that Mr Little had taken out the man's cancerous bladder five years previously. The operation had clearly been a success, for here was the patient and the patient was alive – and talking.

'Good morning Mr Little, I hope you're well. I hope your family is well. I hope that you're not rushed off your feet with people like me needing your attention. The hospital looks busy. Very busy in fact ...

Mr Little wanted to ask the man how well his ileostomy was working.

'You know, Mr Little,' the man continued, 'I couldn't help but notice how busy the hospital looks. There are people everywhere. You must be kept in that operating theatre all night long what with the number of patients that there are around ...'

Mr Little was frowning. He sat forward on his seat and stared at the patient as if willing him to stop talking so that he could get in a question about the functioning of his ileostomy.

'Mr Little, do you remember that time when I was in the wards just after my operation when you had to take me back to theatre because my surgical scar burst open? Goodness me was I poorly, but then you cured me. Sewed everything back together again you did …'

Mr Little was getting irritated. He ground his shoes into the parquet under his desk and scratched his chin. If only the chap would let him get a word in he could finish the clinic promptly and get off to lunch on time.

'Oh yes, you saved my life, Mr Little, and my wife and I are ever so grateful to you, ever so grateful. Have you been outside this morning, Mr Little? The weather's changed something dreadful, you know. Goodness me, it's blowing up something nasty. You'd better wear a hat when you leave the building, it's bound to rain later you know, bound to rain …'

Mr Little had had almost enough of the man. All he needed to know from him was whether or not his ileostomy was working well. He didn't want to hear about the man's wife or the stupid weather. Mr Little flung his pen down on the desk and pushed back in his chair. MacLeod noticed that he had turned very red in the face.

'Gosh, yes, Mr Little, you had better wear a hat. You are going out after clinic, aren't you? You'd be better off, of course, if you were not, but then if you weren't going out, you might be operating instead. What you need, Mr Little, is a nice rest. You do work so hard, and everyone says that you do – that's just it. You need a good holiday, Mr Little, a good holiday.'

Mr Little could bear it no longer. He threw his fountain pen at the wall. Ink spattered against the wall. He roared, shouted,

'Oh, do shut up, man!'

MacLeod almost jumped out of his skin. The patient blanched and sat sharply upright. Mr Little leaned back and stared angrily at the patient who cowered for a moment, and then to MacLeod's amazement said,

'I *am* sorry, Mr Little, my wife tells me I do go on. Yes, I'm very sorry for rambling on. Please do forgive me for blabbering so much. I'm so sorry to be wasting your precious time.'

Mr Little, notably placated and possibly sorry for his outburst, responded,

'Yes, she's right, you do go on, but let's forget about that and concentrate on your ileostomy.'

The mood in the room settled and Mr Little proceeded to ask the relevant questions. Questions answered, the man left the room apologising profusely …

'… for taking up so much of your valuable time, and thank you ever so much, Mr Little, for saving my life all those years ago. I'm forever in your debt.'

Mr Little harrumphed and drew a large tick in the patient's notes.

There was a knock at the door, then silence. Mr Little looked up and said,

'Come.'

The door opened and a clinic nurse ushered the next patient into the clinic room with a sweep of her hand, scuffing the patient as a lion tamer might throw meat to his charge. The patient cowered in the doorway, and the nurse said,

'Go on in, Mr Crowe. It's Mr Little, the consultant. He won't eat you, dear.' But the look on the patient's face suggested that he feared Mr Little might do just that.

Mr Little shuffled through the man's notes.

'**Yes**,' said Mr Little imperiously. 'This'll be one for you, MacLeod.'

Mr Little stared at the patient jittering in the doorway, a man, who, arms crossed over his chest, shoulders bent, stooped to make himself as insignificant as possible in Mr Little's eyes. But he needn't have bothered because, to Mr Little, the man was already insignificant.

'Come and sit down. No, not there man, here. Sit down, on that chair. Not that chair, you fool. Sit, sit. Just there, there's a good fellow. Well done!' Mr Little boomed, and the man subsided in panic in the chair behind Mr Little's desk.

Mr Little turned to MacLeod.

'One for you, I think, MacLeod.'

And MacLeod, not entirely sure what was meant by the phrase, awaited for events to unravel.

'Now, Sir,' continued Mr Little and if ever a 'Sir', could demean rather than elevate, then that 'Sir' encapsulated nothing other than utter condescension.

'You will be very pleased to know, Sir, that we have found out what's been the matter with you. Isn't that good news? You have prostate cancer. There's nothing much to worry about. It's spread to your bones, but I wouldn't bother your little wife with that. Keep it to yourself. I would don't go disturbing the family with the news ...'

The patient blanched and slumped in his chair.

'... Anyway! Jolly good show!' Mr Little noticed that the man had started to quiver with fear.

'Good God, man, brace yourself. Take a hold, won't you?' Mr Little glared at the patient and muttered,

'Extraordinary. Quite extraordinary.' And then, shaking his head with disbelief at such an exhibition of poor moral fibre, Mr Little turned to MacLeod and mumbled,

'Not British, you know.' and continued,

'Now, do pull yourself together, man, and concentrate. Look here, Sir, this clever doctor ...' and Mr Little turned to introduce MacLeod to the man with a wave of his hand that was of such papal grace and beneficence that it was as though he were introducing the man to royalty,

'... is called Dr MacLeod and he's going to make you better. That'll be all from me. You may go ...'

The patient quivered in his seat. Mr Little stared at him with astonishment and frowned.

'You may go now, Sir. Now, if you don't mind. I have patients to see. Very good! Take him in to the next room would you, MacLeod? Good chap. Jolly good. Next patient, Sister.' Mr Little boomed through the closed clinic door, in a voice of such stentorian dimensions that could be used to strip paint, if necessary.

MacLeod helped the patient from his chair, and led him into the adjacent clinic room.

'You all right?'

'I'll be OK; it was just a little bit of a shock, you know.'

'Of course,' said MacLeod, 'but the strange thing is that you will adapt; you will come to terms with things.'

MacLeod was aware of the inadequacy of his comments, but felt almost helpless trying to comfort the man who had been so brutally assaulted with the news of his diagnosis. The patient sniffed, and pulling a bright paisley handkerchief from his pocket, blew his nose vigorously.

'My name's MacLeod, as Mr Little said, and I see from your notes that you are Mr Crowe, and that you're due to start treatment for the cancer. How do you do?'

MacLeod shook the man's hand which, he noticed, was still shaking from the shock of the news given him by Mr Little. Then he told him the basics about prostate cancer and the experimental treatment that he hoped to give him. MacLeod also explained that he would be involved in a clinical trial and that the man would have time to consider whether or not he wished to be take part in the experimental study. Then, giving the patient an information sheet approved by the hospital ethics committee, he made arrangements for the man to attend the hospital's day ward a week later for treatment with the new drug implant.

The patient put on his hat and stood to leave the room. He turned to face MacLeod as he left.

'You know,' he said, 'Mr Little – his bark's worse than his bite. He doesn't mean to be unkind; he'd do anything for his patients. I know he's got a heart of gold underneath all that bluster, it's just that he doesn't like to show it.' And MacLeod, nodding, agreed that the patient was right.

The weekend came, a weekend on call for MacLeod. And although his main duties were on the oncology wards, the occasional referral from other on-call doctors came his way and MacLeod would find that he was summoned to help with newly diagnosed cancer patients on other hospital wards. One referral call took him to the urology wards. MacLeod pushed through the doors into the ward to find the urology ward round in full swing. A line of doctors and nurses were shuffling from bed to bed, checking observation charts and scribbling on prescription sheets. The ward round didn't look quite right, though. It seemed thin; it looked underpopulated. The houseman was there looking weary and stressed, the staff nurses were there looking perky and fresh, the patients were in there beds looking as if nothing was at all wrong with them, looking as if their stay in hospital was a lovely alternative to a Thomas Cook sun-drenched Ibiza holiday. MacLeod approached the round and one of the junior doctors came forward to meet him.

'I've come to see the referral,' said MacLeod with a smile.

'Sure, thanks for coming. I think Mr Miller is on his way to join us. He wanted to introduce the patient to you.'

MacLeod realised then why the urology round seemed underpopulated: there was no Ron Miller on the round. Mr Miller was the senior registrar on the urology firm. And then, as if on cue, Mr Miller roared into the ward with a tremendous crash and clatter of swing doors ricocheting off walls. Ron was wearing full riding gear, jodhpurs billowing, tail coat in a twist, boots muddied, riding helmet tipped dangerously low over his eyes. And Ron was in a sweat.

The houseman gasped, and stuttered quite superfluously, 'Oh, look. He's here!'

Ron marched into the ward and stomping up to the nurses' station, ground his right foot into the floor with a ferocious stamp. Scowling at nobody in particular and everyone in general, he looked around the ward and growled, 'Bastards!'

Ron's eye caught MacLeod and he launched himself towards him, waving a riding whip around his head. The whip came down with a smack onto the nurses' desk. Patient records scattered to the floor. The whip thrashed through the air and its whistle hissed through the wards. Ron crunched towards MacLeod and the floor vibrated.

'MacLeod, you bastard. How are you, old boy? What the hell are you doing here? Shouldn't you be back in that lab of yours?'

MacLeod understood instantly that he was being greeted with considerable friendliness.

'I'm good, thank you, Ron.'

'"Good"? That's not what I heard, my boy. "Bad" is what I heard, mwah, mwah.'

MacLeod wondered why Ron was being so polite. Did he want something from him? Ron slapped his riding whip against his thigh and bellowed,

'Nice to see you. Now what's this I hear about these implants of yours? Sounds very interesting. I'd like to put one in, MacLeod. We've got a patient for you and he's waiting to be treated. So, go to it, MacLeod. Go and get one of those implants from wherever it is you keep the buggers and I'll put it in now.'

'It's not that straightforward, Ron. The patients have to be consented, and they have to be given time to make up their minds whether or not they want to be in the study. You can't just rush them in to an experimental treatment, you know. It's quite a business, Ron. The trial has been approved by the hospital ethics' committee.'

'Ethics! Ethics committee! Bunch of goody-goodies with too much time on their hands. Cause a load of trouble, they do. Know about that sort of rubbish, old boy? It's a joke really. Hmmmph – ethics committee – load of old cobblers, if you ask me. Pity that the bastards don't ask me about bloody ethics, mwah, mwah. S'pose that's a good thing really!

'Now, there's a good boy, MacLeod. Why don't you just run along now and get the implant from wherever it is that you keep the bloody things and I'll shove it in the old bastard.'

'But Ron ...'

'Don't worry, MacLeod, it's fine. Don't you worry at all! It's all completely kosher. It's one of your old boys – he's already been consented by you. The stupid old bastard was due to have his implant around now. Came in through Casualty last night with acute retention. Sorted that out, don't you know. He's a silly old bugger!'

MacLeod looked around the ward and there, sure enough, was his man, Mr Crowe, the patient that he'd met in Mr Little's clinic.

'OK then, Ron. I can see he is one of "mine". I'll go and say hello and then I'll get an implant for him.'

MacLeod went over to Mr Crowe's bed. The man was lying flat on his back, sheets up and over his chin, huge bony nose poking towards the heavens. A plastic tube crept from under the sheets at waist level, and ran down into a transparent plastic bag secured in a plastic stand clipped to the side of the bed. Urine was passing down the catheter tube and trickling into the collecting bag.

'Hello Mr Crowe, how are you?'

'Oh, Doc, how nice to see you. They've looked after me lovely, like.'

'Great. The doctors all think it's about time that you started your treatment. Have you thought about the clinical trial?'

'Yes, I have, Doc. I have thought about it, and we've discussed it at home. I want to do the trial. The family is in agreement that I should go ahead with the new treatment.'

'Great! I'll go off and get the implant and the papers that you'll need to sign. I'll be back in a mo, and then we can get you started.'

'Thank you, Doc. I'm really keen to get going, and then maybe we'll be able to get rid of this ...'

And Mr Crowe tugged disconsolately at his catheter.

MacLeod hurried off the ward to get the implant. He pitied the patients and nurses caught up in the maelstrom of Ron's temper and hoped that he would refrain from whipping the houseman. Once he'd found the implant, he returned to the ward.

'Right, MacLeod, where is the damn thing?'

MacLeod handed Ron the implant. It was about half an inch long and a sixteenth of an inch in diameter, and wrapped in a protective clear plastic sheath. The implant had to be unwrapped and then placed into a hollow needle with a cutting tip. The needle was then attached to a syringe fitted with a plunger that passed through the needle. The needle had to be inserted through the patient's skin, the plunger pushed through the needle, and the implant could then be delivered into the layer of fat beneath the skin. It was an easy, quick and painless procedure. The patient didn't need any local anaesthetic because of the needle's small calibre. All that the patient would notice would be a tiny prick and a pushing sensation as the implant was injected. It was a whole lot better than castration.

Ron looked at the implant and, holding it up to his face, turned it this way and that staring at it with hostility. He tugged at his moustache and growled,

'Harrumph. Bit of a bugger this. Bastard implant. **Nurse**!' Ron shouted and a staff nurse came running to his side.

'Yes, Mr Miller?'

'Lay up a trolley would you, darling, there's a good girl. I want scalpels, stitches, swabs and gloves. And I want local. At once, there's a good girl. Go! Chop, chop. Run! Now!'

MacLeod had ceased to be astonished by Ron's manner some months previously, but did remain amazed at the fact that nurses and junior doctors would take him so seriously as to do as he asked them. It was extraordinary.

The nurse came back within a few minutes pushing a trolley laden with surgical equipment. Ron looked at the trolley angrily.

'Curtains ...' he growled, and the nurse pulled the curtains around Mr Crowe's bed, as Ron stalked off to wash his hands. He returned wearing a face mask, hands held high dripping with water. He stared balefully at the nurse.

'Well! Don't just stand there looking gormless, girl. Open the bloody packet of gloves.'

At this, a terrified Mr Crowe sat up in bed, and pushed his sheets back.

The nurse opened a packet of gloves and tipped them on to a sterile towel unfolded on the trolley.

'Right!' said Ron and flicked on his gloves.

'Ron,' whispered MacLeod. 'You don't really need all this sterile stuff; it's only an injection.'

'Shut up, MacLeod, I know what I am doing. Of course, I need to scrub for this. It's an operation isn't it? For God's sake, man, shut up and let me get on with it.'

Mr Crowe blanched and clenched his fists.

'Now, where's the blasted local anaesthetic? Nurse! **Nurse!** I told you I needed anaesthetic. Where is the blasted stuff? You are bloody useless woman.'

'Sorry, Mr Miller.'

'Ah, that's it. Good show. I'll just squirt some in the blighter.'

Ron launched towards Mr Crowe waving a syringe filled with local anaesthetic, spraying droplets over the bed.

Mr Crowe tensed as Ron ripped back his sheets and pushed back his pyjama top with his elbow. Mr Crowe flinched and juddered back on his pillows.

'Little prick. Hold still, man. Hold still. It's only bloody anaesthetic.'

Ron bent over Mr Crowe, sweat pouring from his forehead and injected lignocaine under the skin of Mr Crowe's belly. Mr Crowe squirmed in terror.

MacLeod held his breath and shook his head. The nurse looked very anxious. Ron threw the anaesthetic syringe onto the surgical trolley and mumbled,

'Where is the damn thing?'

'Nurse! What are you bloody doing, nurse? Pay attention. Scalpel!'

'Ron, you don't need a scalpel.'

'Look, who's in charge of this bloody operation? Is it you, clever boy, or is it me? I think you'll find, MacLeod, that it's me. So just shut up, Professor Smartiepants.'

'**Nurse!** Wipe my brow.'

The staff nurse took a swab from the trolley and dabbed Ron's brow.

'Right.'

Ron waved his scalpel in the air and advanced on Mr Crowe. Mr Crowe cringed with fear and tried to back away. Ron leered at him, scalpel held high and boomed,

'Keep still, you old pouf; you don't want the nurses think-ing you're a faggot, do you?'

Mr Crowe braced himself, his body rigid, arching over the mattress. He groaned. Ron slashed at the area of anaesthe-tised skin. A fleck of blood appeared in the cut.

'Swab – I said **swab,** nurse!' Ron daubed at the wound with a sterile swab.

'Give me the implant, MacLeod.' MacLeod passed the sterile syringe loaded with the implant to Ron and Ron injected the implant through the incision and into Mr Crowe's subcutaneous tissue.

'There. Perfect. Stitch, nurse.'

The stitch was passed to Mr Miller and he sewed the wound's edges together. Ron swabbed the skin clean and with great pomp unfolded an enormous plaster from its packet and, placing it over the wound, turned to Mr Crowe and beaming, said,

'There, you silly old fool. That was easy, wasn't it? Goodness knows why you made such a fuss about a silly little thing like that?'

But Mr Miller might as well as saved his breath because poor Mr Crowe had fainted clean away.

Chapter 9
The Way Home

It had been yet another long duty weekend on call for
MacLeod, a long duty weekend of sustained, sleepless,
exhausting hours in Casualty and completely debilitating
hours on the wards that had begun on Friday morning and
had just come to a close late Monday afternoon. Not the sort
of weekend that exists nowadays except during dark nights in
the City during corporate takeover season.

MacLeod had qualified before the European Work Time
Directive had humanised doctors' working conditions. Today,
in the twenty-first century, it seems inconceivable that anyone
could be made to be on call for the number of consecutive
hours that junior doctors were expected to work only twenty
or thirty years ago.

For MacLeod, the on-call weekend at St Mary's Hospital
had been furiously busy panicky hours overflowing with
blood and pus, and decorated by death and disaster. In the
very few instances that he had managed to escape to the on-
call bedroom and had got into bed, he'd been bleeped out of
his chrysalis of cold sheets, bleeped to come to Casualty,
bleeped to come to the wards. The weekend was about survival – MacLeod's survival.

MacLeod's duty weekend had started on the Friday morning at around 8.30 am with ward rounds and had gone
through to Friday afternoon clinic, continuing with Casualty
calls through Friday night. And then after the Friday night

J. Waxman, *MacLeod's Introduction to Medicine*,
DOI 10.1007/978-1-4471-4522-6_9,
© Springer-Verlag London 2014

take, the white coat parade of the sick and dying, there had been the Saturday morning rounds of the admissions from the night before and then the calls back to Casualty to book in the fresh stroke victims and the new blood clots, the rancid drunks and the green-faced overdoses, the death's door pneumonias and the broken heart attacks.

MacLeod's Saturday afternoon had continued in much the same way as his Friday night and Saturday morning. And then, of course, there was the whole of Saturday and the whole of Sunday, the entirety of sleepless Saturday and Sunday nights. His were midnight's corridors and the clamorous wards; his were the icy lift vestibules and the shuttered pharmacy; his were the heating pipes rattling in a lonely hospital, the loveless wind whispering in an empty outpatient's department.

Medicine was uncivilised in the last century and the juniors acquired their clinical skills through nights and days that were filled with unremitting and extended work. Medicine was a tortured apprenticeship that had to be survived, where experience came riding waves of exhaustion and the clarity of clinical acumen developed during sleepless hours. And good luck to the hapless patient who faced the exhausted junior doctor who'd been up for two nights and two days, the junior doctor whose diagnostic skills had been lost in the labyrinthine empty-headedness and immutable exhaustion that was the consequence of the overwhelming rush of the twenty or so admissions through Casualty and the hundreds of calls from the wards from nursing sisters requesting drips and staff nurses asking for discharge letters, and from registrars querying fluid balance sheets and prescription charts.

By contrast, nursing hours in the same period were limited and sensibly controlled. The nursing hierarchy had ensured a civilised way of life for their juniors. For the nurses, the rush of work stopped and was finite. Their duty rotas had breathing spaces. The nurses worked though eight-hour shifts which included regulated and protected lunch, tea and supper breaks. Woe betide the doctor who ventured into the nurses' office at tea break asking for a patient's temperature chart or for help with a catheter. That tea break was sacrosanct and the doctor would be chased out of the office by raised eyebrows and chilling comments that centred on the inviolate nature of the nurses' duty breaks. Doctors, of course, had no duty breaks, and were unlikely to be offered digestive biscuits and sweet tea in Sister's office at tea break – unless they were dating Sister.

So, MacLeod had been on duty from 8 am on Friday morning until 6 pm on Monday afternoon, with no time off for breathing. He had made it to the lavatory a few times. He looked gaunt, rumpled and hollow eyed – because he *was* gaunt, rumpled and hollow-eyed! There was a certain grey and clammy stickiness to his skin. He had not shaved but he had managed to change his shirt. He was in dire need of vegetables that had not been stewed and a source of calories and minerals that was not draped in polyurethane film. He needed food that had not been camped for two to three weeks in a hospital canteen's freezer cabinet before being zapped in a microwave oven.

MacLeod was looking forward to a beer. He was at that point in the Geneva Convention's Universal Index of Fatigue where there were ghosts in the architecture and paranoia in the furniture. He couldn't think straight. At one point on Sunday afternoon, he'd fallen asleep whilst walking.

The duty weekend agenda rolled seamlessly into a bleary Monday morning and then a stuporous Monday afternoon. MacLeod's head was a useless echoing space and he was the walking dead, struggling through the zombie hours of a working day, but it was a day with an end, an end which meant that he could go home, *home* at the end of Monday afternoon.

Before he could go home, however, MacLeod had to prepare for a ward round, a prowl around the weekend's admissions with an acerbic and hostile consultant and the consultant's host of know-all sleep-in registrars. Organisational skills and charm were needed, if a junior doctor was to make the grade. In zombie mode, MacLeod was quite drained of any of these essential resources that were needed to persuade receptionists to bring forward scan appointments or to manipulate pathology department staff to release test results. He was mentally incapable of flirting sufficiently with the social workers so that the wards would be cleared of the old and the merely homeless and prepared for the next cycle of admissions. Before MacLeod could go home, there were relatives to be spoken to and discharge letters to be written for patients' GPs. Such was the call of duty – a 100 decibel call that howled, shrieked and wailed.

But the weekend duty was at last over and MacLeod was finally free, free to drive home in his little Mini, rust held together by paint. The Mini had 56,000 miles on the clock. By 6 pm on Monday afternoon, MacLeod had around 82 hours at work on his dial. But as he pulled out of the hospital car park, his exhaustion lifted a little, as his responsibility for the near dead and just about living was shed and passed to the new on-call team. MacLeod was escaping in the spring sunlight, on the run from St Mary's Hospital, London W2, ensconced in his little white Mini, coasting along Praed Street in second gear.

MacLeod turned on the radio to the BBC news, voices from another galaxy – the world outside Planet Hospital. In Praed Street, pedestrians passed and Belisha beacons flashed. There were buses and white vans, and the street lights were considering their illumination. And all this went on as though the hospital was nothing; pedestrians walked and beacons flickered as if infection and organ failure did not exist. MacLeod wondered how it was that the world outside the hospital could be so oblivious to its proximity to death's doors, doors to which MacLeod had momentarily held the keys.

MacLeod drew up at the lights at the junction of Praed Street and the Edgware Road. Coming to a halt, he put the car in neutral and pulled on the handbrake. He was so tired that he could only just about manage to see through the mists of exhaustion. It was with effort that he coordinated his legs and his arms as he changed gears, revved and steered. The traffic scooted along the Edgware Road, shuffling and bumbling through the stops and starts of the afternoon rush hour. In the near lane, vans and lorries rumbled north to Kilburn, jostling with commuter cars and the occasional bike, whilst the few desultory vehicles travelling southwards exulted in a journey against the flow of traffic.

MacLeod wound down his window, and spring air embellished with traffic fumes and dust rushed into the car and chased three loose pages of his *A to Z* around and around the interior and back again. Engine idling, MacLeod's exhaustion seemed to lift and he was at peace. He felt that he had done his bit at the hospital and looked forward to chilling out on his musty sofa, sharing the cushions with a nice cup of tea or just possibly a nice cup of beer. There was that good book, and the music system's cool jazz. He was so totally tired that he couldn't really imagine much else.

'Home,' he thought, 'home and maybe after the beer, a nice hot bath and an early night.'

MacLeod's thoughts rattled around in a circuit of inconsequence and ended up without conclusions. The lights changed. He put his car into first gear and crossed the Edgware Road, rumbling along Chapel Street, the little slip road that rustles past the back entrance to Edgware Road tube station. At the T-junction at the end of Chapel Street, he joined a queue of cars waiting to shuffle forwards through the cascade of traffic lights. He shifted into first gear and turned left into the Old Marylebone Road.

MacLeod and his little Mini then approached another set of traffic lights in Old Marylebone Road, lights that blocked his way into the melee of traffic in Marylebone Road. As he slowed to a halt, MacLeod heard the grating and revving of an engine behind him. He glanced up at his rear-view mirror to see the bulge of a Post Office van's bonnet looming over the back of his car. The vehicle was too close. The driver revved his engine again and again, anxious to be off and the van edged forward to leave no air between the van's bumper and the Mini's boot. MacLeod, thinking that the lights were changing, glanced up at the traffic signals. They were still red.

'Goodness that van driver's in a hurry!'

The driver revved his engine again and the van shifted closer.

'Much too close,' thought MacLeod and inched forward, too.

But as MacLeod's Mini moved forward, so too did the Post Office van, mirroring the little car's movements.

'Very, very close,' thought MacLeod. He looked up at the lights but they were still red.

Then, suddenly, the Post Office van's engine roared and the van crunched into the back of the little white Mini, making the most appalling sound.

'Christ! He's hit me!' MacLeod shrieked.

The lights were still red.

MacLeod jumped out of the car, leaving the driver's door open and walked around to the back of his Mini to inspect the damage. As he did so, the van driver reversed giving MacLeod a clear view of the huge, paint-smudged dent in the boot.

'Bugger it!'

MacLeod shook his head in disbelief.

'What a bloody mess! What the Hell has he bloody well done? That'll cost more to fix than the car's bloody worth! What a blasted nuisance!'

MacLeod stormed over to the Post Office van's driver door and looked up at the imbecile. The man had swimming-pool eyes that wobbled behind pebble glasses. His tie was skew-whiff and his collar unbuttoned. He was unshaven and sweaty. The lights changed to green. A chorus of horns beeped and tooted from the line of cars accumulating behind the van.

The van driver wound down his window and leaned out of the cab.

'You went into the back of my car.'

'Sorry, mate.'

The hoots of the car horns ebbed and flowed, crescendoed and died. A couple of drivers got out of their cars for a better view of the crash.

'Why on Earth were you in such a hurry?'

'I wasn't mate. Not in a hurry. Didn't see how close you were to me. It's a small car you've got. Didn't see the back of it, did I? Your car's too bloody small.'

'But that's no excuse for going into the back of me. It's clearly your fault.'

'Yes, mate.'

'We'd better exchange details, then, for the insurance.'

'Yes, mate.'

MacLeod looked down at the dent in his Mini, sucked in his cheeks and tutted like a chicken.

'A weekend on call! This shouldn't have happened! How could this have happened to me?', he despaired.

MacLeod stared up at the van driver, who avoided his gaze and started to whistle. MacLeod noticed that not only was the whistling tuneless but also that it was tasteless. He disliked the van driver.

'So, can I have your name and depot details, please?'

'Yes, mate.' The van driver picked his nose, looked away from Macleod, whistled and then rolled a cigarette.

The sound of hooting picked up again and the clamour got worse.

The van driver withdrew into his cabin and wound the window up so that just the narrowest of gaps was left between him and MacLeod, a gap designed to let in just the tightest of conversational remarks and let out cigarette smoke.

'Look, mate. Why don't we pull over to the other side of the Marylebone Road and get out of their way?'

The van driver's glasses caught the sun and flashed brightly.

'Sure.'

MacLeod walked back to the Mini and clambered in. His little car felt unclean, as if the damage had defiled it and made the Mini a foreign and alien place. He found himself talking to himself muttering.

'Bloody nuisance!' and 'Bloody Post Office van drivers!' and 'Bloody insurance people!' and 'Oh, that's all I bloody need now when I want to get home for a bit of R&R!'

The lights changed again and MacLeod drove across the Marylebone Road turning right towards Euston. He pulled over to let the accelerating queue of cars pass – and pass they did. But the wretched Post Office van passed too, clearing off into the distance, a poisonous disappearing splot of a red van, weaving between the cars, vanishing in the traffic of the Marylebone Road.

'**Bloody Hell**!' MacLeod shook his head in disbelief. 'The bastard! How could he *do* that?'

MacLeod almost felt like crying, but he was a grown man so he limited himself to hitting his steering wheel and cursing in a middle-class, tired sort of a way. The cursing was pretty pathetic.

MacLeod drove home and settled by his phone to call his insurers' office. He got through to his insurance agent, whom he'd dealt with since he was nineteen when he had first started to drive.

'I'm sorry to hear that! Did you have any witnesses?'

MacLeod explained that all the witnesses had driven off down the blasted Marylebone Road in a blasted convoy with the blasted Post Office blasted van.

'Did you get the van driver's details?'

MacLeod explained that he'd been taken in by the van driver's offer to exchange details whilst not blocking the traffic.

'I'm awfully sorry, MacLeod, but if we haven't got the driver's details then the claim's going to be complicated.'

'What do you mean?'

'You're going to lose your no-claims, mate.'

'Oh no!'

'Yup. Better report it to the police. It's a criminal offence you know.'

'What is?'

'Driving away from the scene of an accident. They'd want to prosecute, you know.'

'That's all I need!'

So MacLeod's spot of R&R became a spot of Q&A. After an hour of queuing in the local nick, he gave his details and a description of the crash to a bored, flamboyantly moustachioed desk sergeant who explained that there was no way the police could possibly prosecute a Post Office van driver without more specific information about the man and his van. The police sergeant looked up from his computer screen and asked,

'Do you know how many Post Office van drivers there are in North London, Sir?'

MacLeod assured the sergeant that he had absolutely no idea how many Post Office van drivers there were in North London.

'Sorry, Sir, but that's just the point. That'll be it. Nothing else that we can do, Sir. Sorry. No details, no charge.'

And to emphasise there could be no charge, the sergeant tore off a slip from the Station's Incident Book and gave it to MacLeod for future reference.

'Great!' exclaimed MacLeod as he stumbled out of the station clutching his reference slip.

'Not great at all. It's just rubbish. How could the bastard have done that to me? For goodness' sake! It's not as if it's even his own van. The Post Office would surely have covered the claim. Bloody Hell!'

The number of 'Bloodies' and 'Hells' that littered MacLeod's soliloquy seemed to be increasing with the evening's hours.

'Nothing I can do about it? It's so bloody unfair!'

MacLeod was on the edge of tears. It all seemed so unjust. He drove home from the station feeling so low that it was about all that he could do to get into bed without supper, fully clothed, shoes on. He'd had enough.

But the next day was a different day not just because it was Tuesday rather than a Monday, but because it was a day that followed sleep and with sleep came a renewed zest for life. Once the news got out, all the hospital staff seemed to know of his adventure and all were sympathetic to his plight. On the ward rounds and in the outpatient's clinics, doctors and nurses were united in their view that the van driver was a bad, bad man. As the day passed, MacLeod became more and more determined that he would somehow find the bastard van and get the bastard van driver bastard's details. Details obtained, he would retain his no-claims discount.

In the course of the day, MacLeod came to the view that Post Office drivers probably had rigid work schedules and those schedules were a compound of fixed times and fixed routes. He considered that, with any luck, if he went to the spot where he had his accident and took up his post just before the time of the accident, then he might just get his man.

MacLeod finished work early, handing over to a friend who had wished him luck, and given him a double thumbs-up as he left the building.

So, at precisely 5.45 pm, MacLeod stood poised at the junction of Old Marylebone Road with Marylebone Road, notebook in hand, pen also in hand, and watched the traffic. The stream of vehicles poured over the tarmac as the wind pouted and puffed and made its careless way along Old Marylebone Road ignoring the traffic lights. The reckless wind whistled into Marylebone Road and gusted at the endless flow of cars running west and east.

In Old Marylebone Road, MacLeod had no time for the wind. He only had eyes for the cars as they bore down on him. The wind had no time either for MacLeod but it had time for things of little mass, teasing the leaves and the dust, swirling the sweet wrappers and cigarette foil into housewifely heaps. MacLeod observed that there were blue cars and grey cars, old cars and new pick-up trucks but so far no Post Office vans. He looked at his watch. It was 5.50 pm. The accident had been at 6 pm so there were ten minutes to go if the Post Office van stuck to schedule.

On the street, a tramp bumbled by muttering about demons and drink, whilst office girls hurried home, the clatter of their heels echoes of the passing seconds. The thin sunlight warmed MacLeod's back. He stared at his watch again. It was still 5.50 pm. Not a minute had gone by and neither had the Post Office van. MacLeod counted yellow cars to pass the time, and then he counted Vauxhalls and Fiats. He had not counted cars since his early teens. Then counting cars become a bore and bringing himself to remember the maturity that he was supposed to have, MacLeod thought about his girlfriend instead of the cars, but thinking about his girlfriend took precious little time because he hadn't got a girlfriend to think about.

The wind still blew and the cars still passed and there had been so much blowing and passing that MacLeod considered giving up the search for the Post Office van as a bad job. But steely resolve set in and, as there were still some minutes to go until 6 pm, MacLeod determined to stick to his post. He stood at the traffic lights, a sentry inspecting cars, alert for anything that was red and had wheels. He stuck his hands in his pockets and then took his hands out of his pockets because it was something to do. He whistled and then thought he might sing, but he stopped singing almost as soon as he started because there were two rather fine-looking blondes bearing down on him and he didn't want to appear to be mad because that would not do.

The girls walked passed just as MacLeod exclaimed, to their consternation,

'Hang on … there he is!'

And there he was indeed: hunched over the wheel, floating around a corner, roaring up to the lights, engine revving, exhaust billowing.

Ignoring the girls, which was against his nature, MacLeod implored to the lights,

'Please be red!', and the girls, who now thought he was indeed mad, looked away avoiding eye contact.

But God was on duty that Tuesday afternoon. The lights turned to red and the Post Office van screeched to a halt. MacLeod drew his raincoat around his chest, stood tall, held his stomach in, shrugged his shoulders, and marched in a determined and military fashion into the road. He stomped up to the van driver's cab. The driver looked nonchalantly at him and then looked away and stared straight ahead at the lights.

MacLeod knocked at the window.

The driver lowered the window a jot, and sucked in his cheeks, a cigarette dangling unlit from the corner of his mouth, his face an undergrowth of three-day stubble,

'You bumped into my car yesterday and drove off.'

MacLeod heard his own words and felt the wash of his feeble middle-class upbringing trickle down his trousers.

'Whachatalkinabot, son?'

'You smashed into the back of my Mini yesterday, told me to pull over and then you bloody well pissed off.'

The van driver turned to MacLeod and sneered,

'You're in the middle of the road, son.' The driver's chin wobbled in indignation and his swimming-pool eyes goggled at MacLeod and took note of his trembling. 'Why don't you get out of the way of the traffic, son?'

'That's what you told me to do yesterday. I shan't get out of the way until I've got your details.'

MacLeod peered at the van driver trying to note any identification that he might have, but there was none. No neat number sewn to the man's lapel, no clue to his name. The lights changed, and MacLeod skipped out of the way of the traffic as engines revved and vehicles lurched forward. But he had his notebook open and pen poised to take down the Post Office van's number plate. Job done! MacLeod shuffled away to his car and the phone call to his insurance agent.

'Well done MacLeod! You got the van's details. Fantastic! Did you find any witnesses?'

'Nope. Couldn't ask random drivers if they'd seen the crash yesterday, could I?'

'S'pose not!'

'So, what do you think?'

'I'm sorry, MacLeod but it really doesn't make any difference to the claim. You still stand to lose your no-claims bonus unless the van driver owns up to the accident. Of course, you could try the police and see if they'll press charges. If they do, then your no claims is safe. Why don't you give them a call?'

So MacLeod tried the police, but after an eternity of waiting to be connected was told that there was nothing that the police could do.

'I'm sorry, Sir. It's one person's word against another. You'll understand, Sir, won't you, that there'd be no end of trouble sorting out who's telling the truth?'

MacLeod put down the phone and ruminated about the injustice of the world. So unfair that he'd have to pay for someone else's bad driving. It was pointless calling the Post Office depot, he thought, his word against the driver. Might be worth a try but,

'Dammit, what a waste of time. They'll all stick together, the stinking bastards, bastard Post Office van drivers. I wouldn't stand a chance; there's no point. What's the point in ringing? I can't be buggered to call the depot.'

With this thought occupying most of his mind most of the time, MacLeod got on with his job and got on with his life. The next weekend was his weekend off duty, and he drove his battered Mini to visit Humphrey, his car mechanic. Humphrey's workshop was a lugubrious cave under the railway arches. Bright lights blared and a radio played forgotten tunes. Humphrey's assistant, Bert, spawn of the marriage of an orang-utan and a bearded leather jacket, eighteen stones with a bravura limp, shuffled over, inspected the dent and shook his head.

'It'll cost you!' he shrugged. 'Bad luck mate, bloody bad luck. Wanna cuppa tea mate? We've got the kettle on. **Bert, give 'im a cuppa!**'

Bert shambled over to a hosepipe sitting in a grease-emblazoned bucket of water and filled a saucepan from the hose. He put the saucepan on a camping stove and grinned at MacLeod. Bert's mouth had fewer teeth than the Eiffel Tower.

MacLeod took a chipped grease-smudged mug from Bert and thanked him.

' 'ow many?'

'How many?'

'Sugars, mate?'

'No thanks – this is just great.'

'You'll need to see Jeffrey; he'll sort you out for cash.'

'Thanks Humph, I'll do that.'

And with a recommendation from Humphrey to consider cash only, MacLeod reviewed the dented Mini with Jeffrey who would fix it, he said, for 'notes!' The appointment for the car doctor was duly fixed for MacLeod's next on-call week.

So MacLeod's days passed with their usual routine, the weekly play that is life and death. Hospital life was serious, and MacLeod's work was an engagement with high-powered academic medicine. Medicine at St Mary's was dominated by intellectual dramas such as 'Let's play doctors and nurses!' and 'Hide the stethoscope'. However, MacLeod could not immerse himself in the detail of academic life; his mood had become miserable, his very being was haunted by the insuperable injustice, and this injustice overwhelmed his days. Whatever he did, wherever he was, the sheer awfulness of what had happened to his car seemed to follow and oppress him. Life seemed to him to be very unfair.

'Come on, MacLeod, what's wrong with you?'

'There's nothing wrong with *me*, mate. There's something wrong with my *car* ...'

And to whoever was near, to whoever was prepared to listen, the tale of the Post Office van was recounted and recalled, done over and done to death.

'Sure, mate, it's unfair, but get over it. It's only a car. Nobody was hurt, the car can be fixed.'

'Yes, but it's not fair is it? Not right, the bastard, the bloody van bastard, there's no justice!'

'Look, MacLeod. There's no justice in the world and that's how it is. Get used to it. Get the car fixed and forget about justice, mate. Get on with it.'

And so the days rolled by – morning, afternoon and evening – the little Mini still dented, MacLeod moping and just about enduring on-call duty, bleary nights and days of calls to Casualty, and interminable ward rounds and conversations with relatives of the sick. And then it was Thursday, the day before Friday, and the important reason for noting that Thursday was the day before Friday is that Friday marked the beginning of the sprint to the weekend, a weekend not on duty, a weekend free from life in the hospital. Thursday was an on call for MacLeod, on call tainted with its attendant tortures. MacLeod couldn't wait to be a grown-up doctor, couldn't wait for the ultimate privilege of being allowed to sleep and have a normal working week. What a thought, what an aspiration!

It was a particularly busy Thursday. By 6 pm there had been fifteen admissions through Casualty, each admission requiring attention and each generating myriad tasks that ranged from the treatment of life-threatening medical emergencies, to booking scans, to referral to specialist doctors. But the most difficult of all of the tasks that arose from a patient needing admission was the search for a vacant bed on the wards. Bed occupancy was around 100 %. As a result, for each patient admitted, MacLeod had to find a patient to discharge, a discharge that might not be quite medically opportune. He hated the job.

'Wheel 'em in and run 'em out.' MacLeod mused, sitting for a stolen moment in the Doctors' Mess, feet up on a coffee table attractively smeared with the greasy remnants of last night's poisonous curry.

But MacLeod's feet were not to remain on the table for long: his bleep rang out and the operator told him he was wanted in Casualty.

'That'll make a nice change from being wanted in Casualty!' The operator didn't laugh at MacLeod's rather poor joke.

MacLeod walked through the corridors of the hospital. It was rather a nice walk. The hospital's walls were tiled, the corridors winding, and there were passing parades of Victorian piranha pine doors, wrought-iron work, mahogany handrails, and the occasional dodgy oil painting of some aristocratic patron whose owl eyes seemed to follow MacLeod.

Casualty, where MacLeod was greeted by Sister,

'Another one for you MacLeod! No rest for the wicked!' MacLeod was puzzled by Sister's lack of hostility.

'What did she want?' he wondered.

And Sister continued, 'MacLeod, I think the Casualty Officer wants to discuss the case with you before you go and see the patient.'

'Hi, MacLeod! How are you?'

The casualty officer, Naveed Shah, waved an ECG trace at MacLeod.

'MacLeod! This doesn't look good to me. What do you think?'

MacLeod took up the long pink ECG recording and stared at the squiggles, black tracing burnt onto pink squares framed in white.

It was an easy diagnosis, the ECG showed runs of ventricular tachycardia. The tracing looks like a hyperactive hacksaw blade made ready for a massacre. Ventricular tachycardia is a potentially lethal condition due to a profound electrical conduction abnormality of the heart. The condition can be a precursor to, or the result of, a heart attack, and death is the imminent and very likely consequence of ventricular tachycardia if the tachycardia isn't recognised and treated – and treated urgently.

'VT! He'll have to come in.'

'Yep. Thought so. We've put up a drip. He's on a monitor. Anything you want?'

'A bed and the arrest trolley!'

'Coming up and in the reverse order, Dr MacLeod, Sir!'

MacLeod, the admitting officer, ECG trace dangling and Dr Shah, the Casualty officer, lower jaw dangling, followed by Staff Nurse Murphy, bust dangling, arrest trolley to the fore, hurried through the Casualty ward, curtains billowing in their wake.

MacLeod drew aside the curtains and strode into Casualty cubicle number nine. An unshaven man with pebble glasses sat straight up on the bed, ECG leads all over his chest.

The face looked familiar to MacLeod. All colour ebbed from that familiar face. MacLeod stared intently at the ECG monitor. He paced around the Casualty cubicle. MacLeod waved the pink ECG recording paper trace in the air and the paper made a pretty fluttering sound as it rippled around MacLeod's head.

MacLeod stopped at the end of the man's bed and stared with great intensity at the ECG monitor on duty at the patient's bedside. MacLeod stroked his chin and nodded dramatically at Dr Shah, who stared at MacLeod with great puzzlement. Staff nurse stood patiently by the arrest trolley awaiting instructions from the doctors, ready for MacLeod's requests for the drugs that were needed to treat the patient's ventricular tachycardia. As she waited, she emptied needles and syringes from sterile packaging, tipping them onto the top of the trolley.

Meanwhile, the man with the familiar face gasped and clutched his throat. The trace on the ECG monitor blipped, frothed and zipped.

MacLeod looked from the trace to the patient and took up a drug chart clipped to the bottom of the man's bed. Then he took a pen out of his inside pocket and fiddled with the cap, unscrewed the cap and then screwed it back on the pen. Whereupon he put the pen back in his pocket.

'Haven't we met before?'

'Have we, Doc? Not sure about that?'

The ECG monitor seemed to flatline for a moment.

MacLeod waved the trace in front of the man.

'I'm sure we have met you know ...'

And a puzzled Dr Shah said, 'That's a coincidence. You've met him have you, MacLeod? Where did you meet?'

'I'm not sure,' said MacLeod. 'I think it must have been outside the hospital somewhere, but I am not quite sure precisely where.'

MacLeod turned to the Post Office van driver, 'We have met before, haven't we?' and then stared at the man inquisitively.

'No, Doc, no, I'm sure we haven't met before now. I mean, our worlds don't really collide, you being an educated man, and me a van driver.'

'Oh well,' replied MacLeod, 'my mistake. Could have sworn that we've met before. Funny you should use the word "collide". Collide – you know, I think that word reminds me of something. Oh well, no matter, better get on with things then. We can't leave you any longer without treatment. Don't want you to pop your clogs waiting for treatment whilst we try to sort out where we've met before, do we now?

'Lignocaine, please, Staff Nurse.'

The nurse drew out a glass ampoule of lignocaine from the arrest trolley and it broke open. The crack of the glass as it shattered startled the van driver. Then she drew lignocaine up into the syringe which the patient looked at with some panic. MacLeod wrote the drug's name and dose onto the patient's drug chart and gave it to the nurse. Dr Shah carefully injected the lignocaine into the drip as MacLeod scrutinised the ECG monitor. The arrhythmia settled and the ECG trace assumed a regular and normal rhythm.

'That's much better!' said MacLeod eye-balling the van driver, and the man fell back on his pillows, much relieved.

'But are you *quite* sure that we haven't met before?'

The van driver shook his head emphatically. The ECG monitor trace started to oscillate worryingly.

'Oh well,' said MacLeod, as he left the room. 'My mistake!' He shook his head and, turning to the van driver as he stepped through the curtains, said, 'Looks like you'll be here quite some time ...'

The man was admitted to the wards and over the next few days recuperated from his heart attack. He lay strapped to a cardiac monitor and the zigzag lines of his cardiac trace were there to see for all who passed. And every time that MacLeod walked by his bed, the man's ECG monitor could be seen to react and take fright, its electricity dancing to a bizarre rhythm. With time, the sore heart healed and patient recovered. And before the van driver went home from hospital, it seemed that he was struck by conscience. Well, it was either his conscience or his fear of risking the wrath of the gods by not confessing all.

'I've told 'im, Doc.'

'I beg your pardon?' said MacLeod. 'Told who what?'

'Told me line manager about the prang.'

'At last! Thank you. So, can you give me the details, then?'

MacLeod phoned his insurance broker and explained what had happened.

'Wonderful, MacLeod, just fantastic!' laughed his insurance broker, happy for MacLeod at the outcome. 'What a story, what a coincidence! You won't lose your no claims now! Better call the police and tell them what's happened. Remember, it's an offence to drive away from the scene of an accident.'

MacLeod called the police, explained the van driver's misdemeanour, and the boys in blue duly came to interview the both driver and MacLeod on the ward. While they sat in Sister's office, MacLeod recounted the tale of the runaway Post Office van.

'Would you officers like a cup of tea?' Sister asked coquettishly. Sister had always loved the colour blue. The police sergeant crossed his legs and the constable replied,

'Thanks, love. Six sugars, please.'

'Yes, Doc. That van driver's been a bad, bad boy.' The police sergeant shook his head as he took MacLeod's statement.

It seemed that this was not the driver's only motoring offence and this, taken with a number of his previous trans- gressions, led to his criminal prosecution. MacLeod was called to Court as a witness, and his moments in the witness box caused him great discomfort. He couldn't help but feel sorry for the Post Office van driver, even though the man was a villain and had caused him such great upset. He hated to see the driver up before the bench, and wondered why the case couldn't have been settled without such ghastly conse- quences. The consequences were awful because the van driver not only lost his licence but subsequently lost his job.

Chapter 10
Christmas Day in the Workhouse

Christmas in hospitals can be fun. It's not the worst thing in the world to leave one's family for Christmas Day at the coalface.

But, nonetheless ... please can we go home?

You certainly cannot go home. You're to stay at work, tramping the wards and tramping the corridors, at work in the operating theatres and the canteens, in the pharmacy and the laundry, slaving in the laboratories and in Casualty.

At work!

Under the yellow neon of the long corridors, breathing the disinfectant-tinged air, withering under the glare of formidable nursing Sisters, afloat on Camp coffee, at work.

Nonetheless, despite the grind of work, the ordure of illness, the misery of death and destruction, the overwhelming pestilence of pus and purulence, Christmas Day dusted the workhouse with a patina of seasonal glitter.

And under that dusting of Christmas spirit, the duty nurses and doctors, porters and pharmacists somehow felt a little ennobled by their sacrifice in working the Christmas shift.

In each and every ward, under the fearsome eyes of the strictest of Sisters, there was a houseman. Sister's gaze was serious, for the ward was her domain. The housemen were admitted into her realm under certain terms and the strictest conditions, not least of which was that they were to neither stray nor lurk, for hers were the staff nurses and the ward's floorboards, the pressure dressings and the commodes.

J. Waxman, *MacLeod's Introduction to Medicine*,
DOI 10.1007/978-1-4471-4522-6_10,
© Springer-Verlag London 2014

Today was a special day, a dressing-up day for the housemen. There was not a houseman to be seen in corduroys and button down shirt, not a houseman on parade in polyester and nylon, not a houseman in the house in white coat or theatre gear, nor even in nurses' tights and rubber wear. It was a different sort of a day for the house staff. It was Christmas Day and banished was the houseman's normal attire. For every houseman, there was a lovely uniform.

With synchronicity, sixteen hoary-faced nursing Sisters withdrew into their offices and from the depths of their filing cabinets pulled out their housemen's Christmas outfits. The Father Christmas hat – decorated with ten seasons' dandruff; the Father Christmas uniform – red and occasionally brass-buttoned, fur-trimmed and hinting of flatulence, unwashed in a decade, splattered with turkey fat and red wine, smeared with the accretions of a dozen previous incumbents; the Father Christmas outfit – unfolding in the sisters' arms, ready for each and every newly qualified houseman.

Out into the ward went each nursing sister, Father Christmas outfit on her arm, and there in the open ward, a crooked finger beckoned and her houseman was informed of his fate.

'Here you are, young man, get dressed, there's a good chap. It's the tradition you know. I remember your father did the same thing in his day and didn't grumble. In fact he rather enjoyed it, as I remember.

'Go on, get on with it. Just get on with it, there's a good chap. And you're not to scare my nurses, nor am I to find you molesting them. They are not to be touched. Understand, boy? They are my girls and you will behave.

'Go on! Off with you into the sluice and get changed.

'And then you're to come back into the office for a dry sherry and you'll receive your instructions on the distribution of the Christmas presents to the patients.

'Dressed are you? Stuff that in. And tuck in your top. Tighten your belt. Do your flies up! For goodness' sake!

'That's it. Heaven knows what they're producing in medical school, nowadays.

'Yes, that's right. Blue-wrapped presents for the gentlemen and pink for the ladies.'

It was 11.30 am and on every ward, scrub-faced boys and the occasional girl, just out of medical school, just weeks into their first ward job, dressed in red, padded and stuffed – ho de ho, belt tightened under a pillow belly, goodness me what have you there?, swag bag over their shoulders – were parading past the patients, pale in their beds, near stiffs in stiff sheets. What a day it was, Christmas Day in the workhouse, Noel and Noelle on the wards.

Arms folded, at rest from the drugs trolley, at a distance from the bedpans, the staff nurses watched from the nurses' station as, in each of the hospital's wards, the housemen walked the wards, passing from bed to bed, and stopping in turn at each.

In the warmth of the housemen's beneficence, there were gifts for the patients, gifts taken from a ho, ho, ho sack, slung over a ho, ho, ho shoulder.

For each patient, there was a present, a gift-wrapped something of no significance, the stuff of Christmas crackers but nonetheless a paper-wrapped something that was special for each of the patients, a token of love from somewhere, an acknowledgement of their presence in the infinity of the universe that had condensed to the finite germ-riddled space that was their illness in this hospital and this ward.

For the male patients there was a handshake,

'Here's a little something for you, Sir; compliments of the season.'

And for the females a kiss, an on the cheek dry bones kiss, a nowhere else kiss, delivered with a

'Ho, ho, ho. A happy Christmas, my dear.'

At Bed One on Ward 1.3, MacLeod deposited his Santa sack on the floor and gave Mrs Angel her present. He ducked under the blue-rinsed curls of her perm and kissed her on the cheek.

'Happy Christmas, my dear. Ho, ho, ho!'

Mrs A shook MacLeod's hand. MacLeod grinned. He liked Mrs A and was pleased to give her a present. MacLeod felt good. He had done good.

MacLeod shuffled along to Bed Two dragging his goodie bag along the floor. MacLeod reached deep inside and found a present for Miss Goldstein. Miss G, in flannelette and shawl, smiled up at MacLeod and touched her fingers to her lips in maidenly modesty. MacLeod kissed Miss G on her cheek and a ripple of face powder trickled to the sheets.

'Happy Christmas, my dear. Ho, ho, ho!'

MacLeod heaved his bag up from the ward floor, swung it over his shoulder and shuffled along to Bed Three.

Two nurses watched from their station, a desk in the middle of the ward. Leaning back against the desk, their bottoms resting on its edge, arms folded, shoulder to shoulder, legs crossed, they observed MacLeod's progress from bed to bed.

MacLeod was full of fun but at Bed Three, Mrs Frances Clarke's bed, MacLeod's fun tank drained to empty. MacLeod's cheeks paled and his grin slipped to the floor. MacLeod panted, MacLeod felt sick. MacLeod put down his Santa sack and waited for salvation.

Mrs Frances Clarke had been referred to hospital by her GP for investigation of a mysterious illness. Mrs Clarke had been admitted to the wards with bizarre symptoms. She had chest pains and a funny rash. Her memory had gone and the neurologists had been very interested in the spectacular galaxy of cranial nerve changes that manifested in asymmetric pupils and the loss of sensation in her limbs.

Mrs Clarke's hair was an unnatural auburn. Her cheeks hung from high bones and her breasts, under her lavender polyester nightie, were unnaturally pointy.

Mrs Frances Clarke lay wan and worn amidst the starched sheets of Bed Three. Turning her head from side to side, Mrs Frances Clarke puzzled at the Christmas fuss that energised the ward.

Mrs Clarke noticed MacLeod, looked up at him and smiled. The smile was querulous, questioning, a smile that would have been more at home late at night under the shimmering streetlight of Portsmouth's docklands, a diffident smile that seemed to not quite place the nervous-looking Father Christmas who stared down at her.

Mrs Clarke had seen MacLeod and his swag bag. Mrs Clarke had spotted MacLeod kissing Mrs Angel and Mrs Clarke had watched MacLeod kissing Miss Goldstein.

MacLeod contemplated Mrs Clarke as she primped her hair and was alarmed.

Now, Mrs Frances Clarke's Mr Arthur Clarke was a merchant seaman, a seaman adrift on far stormy oceans for long periods in foreign parts.

Rum, bum, sodomy and the lash. It was a sailor's life in the Merchant Navy and a man's life at sea. And how poor Mrs Clarke had suffered from her husband's seafaring ways. Her lips had touched her husband's lips and her husband's lips had touched the purple places where the spirochete frolicked, on wild shores behind the closed doors of the rococo palaces of tainted whores.

So, the puzzling nature of Mrs Clarke's illness had led to the instigation of certain tests that were more usually carried out in the 'Special' Clinic. And these tests had revealed her to have syphilis.

At the nurses' station, two staff nurses observed MacLeod hesitating before Mrs Clarke's bed. As MacLeod hesitated, Staff Nurses Christine Aldag and Josephine Norton simultaneously took in a sharp breath. They tensed inside their stiff, starched, blue and white striped nurses' uniforms. Tall white hats, pinned to their hair, uniforms nipped at the waists by a red belt for S/N Aldag and a blue belt for S/N Norton, black stockinged nurses.

Sister glared and the nurses pretended to busy themselves with reports and forms.

Mrs Clarke was due to begin a course of high-dose intramuscular penicillin. She was to start treatment when all of her tests were completed and completion day was the day after Boxing Day. The delay in starting her treatment was because it was impossible to complete complex medical tests over the Christmas period when the laboratories were running an emergency service only. The consultants wanted to be completely sure about a diagnosis concerning which no one else had the slightest doubt.

In the yellow-tinged ward light, a hesitant MacLeod stood at the head of Mrs Frances Clarke's bed.

The nurses stared at MacLeod and Mrs Frances Clarke, imagining the consequences of that Christmas kiss.

MacLeod and Mrs Clarke. Face to face in the ward. MacLeod leaning awkwardly away from Mrs Clarke, Mrs Clarke stretching yearningly towards MacLeod. And as the colour drained from MacLeod, so blood seemed to suffuse the face of Mrs Clarke, and she became quite rosy faced, aglow with the anticipation of her Christmas kiss.

Oh, how Mrs Clarke wanted a kiss, a kiss just like the ones that MacLeod had given that bitch Mrs Angel and that skinny devil Miss Goldstein. Just a little kiss, a teensy-weensy kiss, that was all that she wanted, only one kiss, a Christmas kiss. The whole ward was to be kissed, so why shouldn't she be kissed by this nice young doctor? It was only fair. And it was her turn for a kiss. 'So,' she thought, 'come along, doctor and give me that kiss.'

Mrs Clarke sat up in bed and drew the sash tightly around her dressing gown. She straightened her bed sheets.

MacLeod stared at Mrs Clarke and took a pace backwards.

MacLeod gulped and turned to pull Mrs Clarke's present from his bag. Mrs Clarke sat up straight in the bed and thrust out her bosom. Mrs Clarke's lips puckered in expectation of a kiss. It had been a long time since she had kissed a young man and she yearned for her kiss.

MacLeod's lips receded into the depths of his mouth.

Mrs Clarke leaned forward, pulled herself up from her pillow and plumped up her hair.

MacLeod's lips retracted into his throat.

Mrs Clarke craned her neck towards MacLeod and MacLeod took a second step back from the bed.

MacLeod turned to the nurses' station seeking help. Staff Nurses Aldag and Norton waved at him.

Sister coughed.

Mrs Clarke's lips were a red, red rosebud and her arms were open for MacLeod and that Christmas kiss.

Brrrrrrrrrrrrrrrrring!   **Brrrrrrrrrrrrrrrrring!**
Brrrrrrrrrrrrrrrrring!
Cardiac arrest Ward 1.2
Arrest. All duty doctors to Ward 1.2.

And MacLeod, snatched from the spirochete's jaws, rushed out of the ward and along the corridor to the arrest in Ward 1.2.

No fewer than eight Father Christmases were clustered around a single bed in Ward 1.2. The bed sheets were stripped back and an unconscious patient stripped to the waist, limbs akimbo, lay stretched out on rumpled sheets. The arrest trolley was at the side of the bed. Dr Ian Radford stood at the foot of the bed. And all around the bed on either side of Dr Radford there were little Father Christmases, big Father Christmases and medium-sized Father Christmases. All the Father Christmases were busy at work, bent over the patient, inserting drips, intubating, drawing up drugs, calling for porters and attempting cardiac massage.

Dr Ian Radford was in charge of the assembled festive throng. Ian was known as Colonel Spanker to his friends, and was named after a retired army officer. The original Colonel Spanker had left the Coldstream Guards and settled in the Sussex countryside, where he took up a hobby, as military men sometimes do upon leaving the forces. But Spanker's hobby had brought him unwanted national attention. He'd become infamous for his spanking activities in Midhurst. He, the 'Sussex Colonel', had been caught in flagrante in a police raid on Madam Whiplash's House of Correction. The colonel had found a sort of fame in the law courts and a nickname in the tabloids. It is not clear why Ian Radford was called Colonel Spanker by his friends, but the nickname did somehow suit him.

Spanker was in charge of the cardiac arrest because he was the senior of the junior doctors on duty. Spanker had a puckish beard, elfin face and unnaturally curled hair. He was a muscular fellow who had crossed the Atlantic, single-handed in a small yacht, the happiest days of his life. And he'd liked the journey so much that he'd sailed the Atlantic again and again.

At University College Hospital, it was traditional for the most senior of the junior doctors to dress in a ceremonial fairy costume on Christmas Day. The outfit was 'nice' and Spanker flaunted it. He wore with pride those white ballet pumps and silver tights, that gorgeous white tutu and the queen of all sparkling tiaras. Spanker had a wand, of course, a wand that was tipped with a glistening diamante clustered star. Spanker's tutu flared out in a pretty curve over bulging thighs. Spanker had inserted a large codpiece in his tights to set off his costume.

Spanker liked his outfit and, in particular, rejoiced in his wand, a wand that a few moments earlier in the day had been used to bless the nurses, a curious ritual that had involved the wand delving into parts of the nurses' outfits that wands were generally banned for exploring.

As Spanker had toured the wards on Christmas patrol, he had attracted a swelling and excited retinue of doctors, and the jollity of the medics knew no bounds. In many ways, the coming together of the giggling gang was to the cardiac arrest patient's advantage because pretty much all the doctors on duty in the hospital had been gathered round Spanker in the adjacent ward when the cardiac bleeps had gone off. At the shrill call of the arrest, the gang of Father Christmases had rushed after Spanker to the arrest and had got to the patient's bedside within seconds of the arrest call.

MacLeod, summoned by his bleep, snatched from the arms of Mrs Frances Clarke, raced from the ward to join the Father Christmases on arrest duty.

So, there were nine Father Christmases now lined up around the bed.

Dr Radford stood at the foot of the bed, wand raised, conducting the arrest, for he was the senior doctor and therefore in charge.

'Get that line in. What are you doing, Man? Get it in. If you can't get it in, let someone else have a go!'

'Anyone know anything about the patient?'

'Yes, came in this morning with chest pain. Admitted through Casualty, the name's James Chubb.'

'Chest compression. Come on!'

'Bicarb. Get the bicarb going!'

'Intubate – for bollocks' sake, get the bugger intubated ...'

'Who's sorting out the bloody defribillator? Who, for heaven's sake?'

'OK. Stand back.'

'Paddles on.'

The anaesthetist placed the defibrillator paddles on the unconscious patient's chest and awaited Spanker's instructions.

'Everyone back!'

The Father Christmases withdrew two paces, and, as one, crossed their arms.

'OK, Chief. Take aim.' Spanker's wand was raised high in the air pointing over the head of the anaesthetist.

Nine Father Christmases gathered in a neat arc around the patient's bed, and there was a fairy at the white and silver apex of that arc of red.

Spanker gesticulated in the direction of the unconscious patient, waved the wand round and around the man's feet and with a flick of the wand commanded,

'Defibrillate. Now! Fire!'

CRUMP. The defibrillator flicked into action and the patient bucked under the shock. And woke up.

The patient lay back in his bed and opened one eye. Just the one eye.

He woke, craned open that eye and saw at the foot of his bed a rather large fairy, a fairy with a wand and a tutu and a tiara. A rather hairy fairy.

The resuscitated man's single opened eye contemplated Spanker and that eye did not like what it saw. The eye bulged. The eye reddened.

The resuscitated man's right hand grasped at his endotracheal tube and yanked it out.

He sat bolt upright.

Terrified.

He roared.

'Crikey!' he gasped, 'I'm in heaven.'

And collapsed back on his pillows, away with the fairies in a dead faint.

But he came round eventually, and to this day, a certain Mr James Chubb of Islington, London, N1 believes in fairies.

Chapter 11
Chutney Wars

Whistling tunelessly, hands deep in pockets full of holes, MacLeod meandered through the outpatient's clinic, a land of peeling paint and uncomfortable seating arrangements. Outpatient's had become a habit but it was a habit that he enjoyed. Outpatient's duties were a pleasure because the patients were mostly well, and always immeasurably grateful for the care they had been given on the wards. It was a cheerful clinic, a celebration of life's victory over death. The patients had been through the worst of experiences, surviving chemotherapy and their cancers. The patients' appointments with the doctors were mostly taken up with family news and monsoon-like outpourings of gratitude. In this clinic, sitting behind an Edwardian oak desk, MacLeod felt as though his medical skills were redefined and had become those of a certain class of old fashioned GP working on remote Scottish islands.

The young doctor had introduced a few of his clinical trial patients into the outpatient's clinic, much to the disapproval of his seniors who wondered what the hell he was doing running his own patients through their empire.

The nurses who ran the clinics were cheery and middle aged; they were experienced women who had worked on the oncology wards and understood what the patients had been through. They were sweet women, ready with a cup of tea and a supply of biscuits brought in from home, sustenance for their doctors. MacLeod entered his clinic room and opened

J. Waxman, *MacLeod's Introduction to Medicine*,
DOI 10.1007/978-1-4471-4522-6_11,
© Springer-Verlag London 2014

the top right-hand corner of his desk, and there, tightly
wrapped in clingfilm was a poppy seed encrusted ham and
salad roll. The roll was a present from Min, who was
MacLeod's favourite nurse. MacLeod loved her kindness,
loved her smiling face. Min was slightly round and slightly
Irish, her hair a tight perm. Min came wrapped as tightly in
her uniform as MacLeod's roll was swaddled in clingfilm.
MacLeod's love for Min was sort of requited love, because
Min loved MacLeod on behalf of her teenage daughter.

MacLeod unwrapped his roll and walked out into the corridor. The outpatient's clinic rooms branched off the corridor
which led out to a cluttered waiting area where a large clock
reminded the waiting patients of the limits to time. There
were six consulting rooms, mostly poky and generally shabby,
and they were occupied by one consultant who resided in the
grandest of the rooms, three registrars, a locum and MacLeod.
At this point in the morning, all the doors to the consulting
rooms were closed except for the doors to MacLeod's and the
locum's rooms. MacLeod gobbling his roll, poppy seeds spilling on the grey linoleum, came to a halt at a twist in the corridor and stood next to a long scabby table on which were
piled the waiting patients' clinical records, soft folders of A4
paper that told of their lives.

Oblivious to everything except for his roll and the
patients' notes, MacLeod stooped over the table and shuffled through the pile of folders. The notes were arranged in
order. At the top of the pile were the notes of the patients
who had been waiting the longest and were to be seen first
by the doctors. Naughty unsporting MacLeod, instead of taking the top set of notes, he shuffled through the pile of
patients' notes looking for the familiar names of patients
whom he had seen and for any patient who might be suitable
for clinical trials of any of the new drugs that he was
researching. But as he searched, MacLeod was unaware of
the soft pad of approaching danger, for stalking silently
towards him, softly, softly, came Dr Ludlow, the consultant in
charge of the clinic. And as he flicked through the notes
searching for 'interesting' patients, naughty MacLeod was

unaware that his consultant loomed behind him, puffed with rage, boiling eyed, bale and bile bubbling. MacLeod was concentrating on the patients' histories, insensible of the cauldron of suspicion bubbling behind him.

"**MacLeod!**" Dr Ludlow boomed.

MacLeod froze, and then defrosting, turned around for a view of an incandescent Dr Ludlow. Although objectively there was no doubt that Dr Ludlow was indisputably the most junior consultant on the firm, from a subjective viewpoint Dr Ludlow was entirely confident that he was the most senior physician. Dr Ludlow had been appointed to his consultancy at the age of thirty. He was old school, Winchester and Cambridge, the right sort of family background, the right sort of leather-patched tweed jacket, his bristlingly shiny brown brogues a paragon of polish.

Dr Ludlow had been a houseman on the medical firm that he now commanded. On entry into medical school at the age of nineteen, Ludlow was already considered an old fogey. As a houseman, he comported himself as a consultant. In the first weeks of his houseman years, Dr Ludlow was entrusted with bearing the flag for propriety by Professor Bodley, the senior consultant on the firm. Professor Bodley was a remnant of Edwardian times, austere, aloof, draped in black gabardine, the last person in London to wear detachable stiff collars. And when Professor Bodley noticed that the senior registrar's hair was a little too long, taking Ludlow aside, Professor Bodley had whispered,

'Ludlow, do tell the senior registrar to get a haircut, there's a good chap.'

When Dr Ludlow became a consultant, he remained in school prefect mode and maintained order on the wards by divine right. He upheld standards, and exploded into a fugue of fury and temper if things were not quite to standard. No sloppiness was allowed on Dr Ludlow's ward rounds, and if a result was missing from a patient's files or if there was a delay in ordering a scan, the volcano that was Dr Ludlow's temper erupted, raining vitriol and brimstones.

Dr Ludlow's twice-weekly ward rounds were held in the patients' sitting room. When the time came for his rounds, the patients, ill and immobile, anaemic and septic, were shooed out of their sitting room by the nurses, drip stands trailing. The TV was switched off and the medical staff shuffled in and took their places – the most senior man and all of the women sitting, the juniors and the rest of the male staff standing. Sister sat at the apex of the ward round, her arms crossed, her smile beatific, and next to her sat Dr Ludlow, eyes crossed, arms waving in a cataclysm of diabolic fury.

Dr Ludlow and Sister Smallpox reigned amongst a garrison of juniors, the king and queen of ward rounds. Each round began with the most junior of the doctors recounting the patients' individual clinical histories in turn to Dr Ludlow. The junior's voice trembled and quaked in expectation of coruscating criticism. During the round, notes were thrown and tears were shed. The patients' histories were related in strict order of the hospital bed number that they occupied. It was considered a major victory if the houseman managed to get half-way through the notes without Dr Ludlow stomping out of the sitting room in a fury of flailing arms. Sitting bolt upright, his mood a maelstrom of malevolence, Dr Ludlow listened to the houseman, his eyes narrowed, his face sizzling with scowls, waiting for faults. When those faults in patient management came, and come they invariably would, Dr Ludlow would bellow with rage, and his furious roaring made the juniors twitch with fright.

MacLeod took part in the ward round as an observer with no active role. There was no choice but to attend, even though he had no ward duties. Attendance was obligatory to all research staff and their presence puffed up the ward round numbers and inflated its importance.

MacLeod's best friend on the wards was Ludmilla Neudachin. Ludmilla had been brought up in Russia, but had been educated in the English educational system, and qualified at Oxford. Ludmilla was indomitable and found all of life amusing. In ward rounds, she was granted the privilege of a seat by virtue of her chromosomes. Settling into the cosiness of one of the patient's armchairs, Ludmilla first stretched, then yawned and, making herself very comfortable, fell asleep. In Dralon's soft embrace, Ludmilla snored gently, her breath keeping time with her billowing bosom. Ludmilla's snoring continued through the storm of Dr Ludlow's tantrums. She was oblivious to the thwack of patients' notes hitting walls, careless of the tearing apart of X-rays, ignorant of the ripping-up of blood test results, and absolutely unaware of the demented demands to get the so-and-so blasted bastard radiologist/haematologist here at once to explain himself. Through the raging of Dr Ludlow's thunder, insensible of his shouting and roaring, deadened to his demands and threats, Ludmilla slept on. MacLeod quizzed her on her behaviour.

'How can you sleep through all that noise and fury, Ludmilla?'

'My dear,' she explained, 'how could I possibly take him seriously? He has such a big bottom.'

With the benefit of this explanation, MacLeod understood why it was that Ludmilla was able to fall asleep in ward rounds.

And it was the same Dr Ludlow who was now looming behind MacLeod, wondering why MacLeod was taking notes from the middle rather than the top of the pile. Aware of vinous breath on his collar, MacLeod turned to Dr Ludlow and grinned, but his grin faded under the scalding opprobrium of Dr Ludlow's scowl. Caught in the act MacLeod, defended himself ...

'Just window shopping, Dr Ludlow!'

... and he put the illicitly taken queue-jumped notes back in their place in the stack. Reluctantly, he then took the first set of notes from the pile and walked along the corridor to his room. As he did so, MacLeod glanced into the waiting area and saw that there were many more patients than usual waiting to be seen and pondered why there was such a queue.

'With a pile of notes that high, it's no wonder,' he thought, 'that Dr Ludlow's on the prowl.'

As he walked past the locum's room, MacLeod had a view through the open doorway of Dr Beetles, the locum, chatting on the phone, head back, feet up on the desk. Dr Beetles was laughing. He was around 30 years old and very bald, his baldness compensated by hugely bushy and unnecessarily long sideburns. Dr Beetles glanced up as MacLeod looked in and nodded amiably. MacLeod waved a greeting and wandered on. He stopped at the next bend of the corridor, his path blocked by a tall West Indian nurse. Fenella's arms were folded across her chest, her usual calm rippled by a thick crease of concern that twitched across her forehead.

'Morning, Fenella. Clinic's slow today, Fenella?'

'Sure thing, doctor … it's *that* locum man. He's not doing nothin', just sittin' there, sittin' there chit chattin' to his friends on the 'ospital phone. I ask you. How we goin' to get through the clinic today?'

Fenella shook her head. 'Dr MacLeod; why's that Dr Beetles not seeing patients?'

'I don't know!' said MacLeod. 'You tell me! Why isn't he seeing patients, Fenella?'

Fenella sighed. 'That doctor, he done tell me that locums don' see patients in clinic. He tell me "Staff Nurse! Patients seen by regular staff only, never locums."'

MacLeod giggled, walked into the clinic room and got on with reviewing the patients in the order that the pile of notes dictated. In time, he came to the patient whose notes Dr Ludlow had caught him looking at. There was a knock on his door.

'Hello Mr Bailey. Come on in.'

The door pushed open tentatively and Mr Bailey peered around the door frame.

'Come through, come in, Mr Bailey.'

Mr Bailey wore a pork pie hat parked at a very rakish angle and he tipped his hat to MacLeod as he entered the clinic room. There were gold chains draped around his neck and wrists. He had on two-tone shoes, and a long stiff raincoat, which drifted open to reveal a white suit, black shirt and a broad, brightly painted tie.

'Hello, Sir.'

'You don't need to call me "sir". Call me "doctor", if you'd like to call me anything. My name's MacLeod.'

'OK, Sir, Doctor.'

'Now, Mr Bailey. How have you been?'

'Me good, Doc.'

'Excellent. And those aches and pains – how are they?'

'Well, me got the pain patch on and I OK, Sir.'

'Great news. It's really good that the pain is under control at last. Now, what do you think about joining the clinical trial that I mentioned to you last week?'

MacLeod had been trying to recruit patients to a clinical trial of a new treatment for prostate cancer. This new treatment was taken as a tablet four times each day. So far, there had been no side-effects from the treatment and there was every indication that the tablets were working; the patients seemed to be getting better. But Mr Bailey had a problem and that problem was that he didn't like taking pills. He couldn't swallow tablets. He'd explained the situation to MacLeod in outpatient's a week previously:

'Tablets, Doc, I no good at tablets. Me gag, me throw up.'

'So you can't swallow them without retching? That's no good is it? Now you mustn't worry, Mr Bailey.'

At the mention of the word 'worry', Mr Bailey had sat bolt upright in his chair, his face registering panic. MacLeod had continued, trying to reassure his patient.

'Please don't worry, Mr Bailey. But do listen to this please. If you feel that you can manage to take the pills, then that's great; all's well and good. But if you can't swallow them, then I'm sorry but you can't be treated in the clinical trial. That's because the new treatment is only available in tablet form.

'But it's OK, Mr Bailey. If you can't manage the pills, then we'll just have to sort out another way of treating you. Now, this is what I want you to do.'

MacLeod remembered that he had leaned forward and put his elbow on the desk that separated him from his patient to emphasise his point.

'Mr Bailey, what I want you to do is this, please. Have a think about the pills. Think about whether or not you can manage to swallow them. See how you get on over the next week. When we meet in outpatient's again, we'll see if you feel that you'll be able to swallow the tablets.'

That had been the situation in the clinic last week and MacLeod was waiting to hear from Mr Bailey how he thought he might manage with the clinical trial tablets.

Mr Bailey leaned forward in the clinic chair and stared at MacLeod, who noticed how beautifully Mr Bailey's shoes had been polished and how immaculately his trousers had been pressed. Mr Bailey looked away from MacLeod and then spoke.

'Well, Doc, me been givin' a good thought to the tablets. Know what I do?'

MacLeod nodded encouragingly as if to imply to Mr Bailey that he knew exactly what he had done. But, of course, MacLeod had not the slightest idea what Mr Bailey had been up to.

'Go on, Mr Bailey. What did you do?'

'Well, Doc, you know me don' like takin' tablets. Them tablets they make me gag, they stick in me throat and me throw up. Well, what me do, see, me practice in me wife's tablets, the blood pressure pills. When Mrs B she take them, me do take them, too and know what, Doc, together we get along fine. Me take her pills and she take the pills and I surprised. All go well. Mind you, Doc. Know what 'appen – new ting, me do feel bit dizzy.'

MacLeod was not surprised that Mr Bailey felt dizzy. Most people with normal blood pressure would feel a bit dizzy taking tablets that put their blood pressure down so low that the blood wouldn't get to their brains.

'You have stopped taking her pills now though, haven't you?'

'Yes, Doc.'

'Good.'

And MacLeod explained again about the clinical trial, and told him never again to take pills prescribed for his wife.

The clinic ended and MacLeod returned to the registrar's office and began to write a review for publication of advances in his area of research. He thought he'd write as much as he could and then return home to change. MacLeod was looking forward to the night ahead. Tonight was Friday night and not just an ordinary Friday night. It was a **Friday Night Special**, the night of the medical school Running Club's annual dinner, which was being held at the Paradise Curry House in Paddington and was sure to be a great evening. It was going to be a Boys' Night Out – fun and laced with lager and curry.

MacLeod wasn't a particularly good runner, nor did he have much sympathy with the concept of involvement in any sporting activity other than sex. His antipathy for any species of organised games had started at school, where in the spring and winter terms there had been compulsory Wednesday afternoon cross-country running. MacLeod tolerated the summer term's cricket which mostly involved a restful time sitting down fielding in the long grass, but running for him had been quite out of the question. As a result, he had confined his sports' activities at school to cross-country walking and resting in the long grass.

Every student at the medical school was encouraged to participate in some form of sporting activity. And for some reason MacLeod had been invited by the Running Club members to be their president.

The Paradise Curry House was entirely as one might imagine it to be. The restaurant was a shady den lined with red flock wallpaper, nestling in a Paddington back street between the Pig and Poultice and the Sir Alexander Fleming public houses, its dull lights twinkling an energy-saving welcome to all. MacLeod pushed through the restaurant doors. Inside, lonely tables laden with stainless-steel chutney pots perched on a tandoori-stained carpet. A mirrored pine-clad bar with a single lager pump reflected MacLeod's image as he took his place at the table reserved for the Running Club. On the restaurant's walls were photographs of pouting, bare-bellied Indian dancers and a painting on brown velvet of the Taj Mahal.

The Running Club's annual dinner had 'Scotland' as its theme. All the club members wore kilts and a bagpipe player had been hired for the evening to pipe the members to a long table in the centre of the restaurant. By the time MacLeod arrived, everyone else had taken their places at the table. 'Scotland the Brave' took him to his seat at the top of the table. He hoped that he wouldn't have to make a speech. The Running Club members looked to a man as though the restaurant had not been their first port of call that the evening. They were all in that stage of giggling tipsiness where everything was fun and nothing was of consequence. Lagers were at hand and poppadom crumbs decorated their sporrans. The waiters loitered behind the bar looking on anxiously.

Outside the restaurant, an ambulance screamed by, siren howling and in answer came the echoing wail of a police car whizzing past at high speed. Inside the restaurant the head waiter stood to attention at the foot of the table, order book open, waiting for the guests to make their choices. But the Running Club boys were overwhelmed by an epidemic of giggling and back slapping and were incapable of ordering their food. MacLeod took responsibility, knowing that the selection of dishes ordered would be largely irrelevant, given the state of intoxication of the diners. He chose a selection of curries and pilau rice, held steady on the vegetables, and asked for sufficient nan bread for all, hoping against hope that the club members would resist all urges to start a bread fight.

There were around twenty men at the table – but unfortunately no women to moderate their behaviour. With a shout, more lagers were called for and trays of frothy drinks arrived courtesy of an anxious waiter. Dishes of curry and rice were served and there was silence at the table as the runners focused on their grub.

MacLeod looked at the faces of the medical students, happy boys, uniform products of the middle classes that fill the vocational courses of the select universities with their children. MacLeod stared at them, and hoped that he wasn't as they were, but he knew in his heart that he was. Life in medical school was the property of the privileged. All the boys were tall. All had clear complexions, and if it were not for their different hair colour and the slightly different jut of their jaws, they could all have been brothers. But pity the mother of these Running Club brothers, when two of her boys decided it would be fun to get under the table and crawled around tying shoelaces to table legs and other shoelaces to unrelated laces. And pity the father of the Running Club family when the inevitable first spoonful of pilau rice was flicked from one end to another of the curry-stained table. The waiters suddenly ducked below the bar as the chutney wars began. Rice spattered the hair of a ginger runner and, in retaliation, a bread ball basted in curry sauce was flicked onto the nose of an innocent blond boy who was not the perpetrator of the original crime.

MacLeod stood up and shouted for order but in response the Running Club cheered him and took no notice of his demand. Undeterred, MacLeod continued,

'Come on, guys, quieten down. Come on, sit down, everyone. Sit down, please.'

At last, the Running Club quietened down, the boys settled into their seats and there was peace for a few moments. The waiters scurried out from behind the bar, and clustered timidly around the serving hatch awaiting deliveries from the kitchens. Then the waiters converged on the table placing stainless-steel plates in front of the runners. There was silence in the restaurant as the runners helped themselves to tandoori mixed grills. Spicy mince kebabs, chicken and lamb chops were piled onto their plates and buried under rice. The silence was punctuated by the chomping of perfect dentition, and then after a lapse of seconds, appetites dampened, the even rhythm of the chomping was shattered by a baritone chant for …

'Lager, Lager, Lager!'

And the rumble of their hymn for lager would not be assuaged until the waiters came rolling in with a tide of more trays of beer.

'More lager!'

The head waiter seemed to pale as he anxiously surveyed the unruly boys. He clasped his fingers, then loosening the top two buttons of his black polo-necked shirt, glanced from the medical school runners to the clock. He was hoping for turning out time without too many upset tables and broken chairs. He wasn't too worried about the stainless-steel plates, a useful precaution for group outings from the medical school.

And now it was joke-telling time. Everyone silent whilst they took turns, and at each punch line, glasses were raised in good cheer, cheer for the joke, cheer for the Running Club and cheer for this and that vestal virgin deflowered on a dusky night, on a moonlit Paddington shore. The Running Club members were enjoying themselves; more beers were called for and more toasts were raised until the moment came for a mass exit to the gents when laces pulled at table legs and runners fell and dinner tables collapsed. But the runners clambered to their feet giggling, for this was considered jolly good fun by all except the waiters, who congregating by the lager pump, decided it was closing time and dimmed the lights once then twice.

The Running Club emerged from the gents in the half light swaying a little, and clutching at each other for anchorage – for they were the Running Club and this was their night out. This was fun and what could be more fun than a night out with the boys? MacLeod noticed that the Running Club captain was talking conspiratorially to the vice-captain, his hand a shield for his garlic-laden mumbling. They nodded at each other and grinned; an agreement had been reached.

The Running Club captain walked over to the head waiter,

'Look here, old boy, you know that we are the Running Club, don't you. Well, it's club tradition …

At that point, MacLeod concluded that he'd really had enough of the evening. He felt that time was up and duty had been done. So, he tossed £30 on the table, his contribution to the expenses of the meal, and deaf to chatter, made for the door of the restaurant as the Running Club captain continued his conversation with the head waiter,

'… for us to race round the block – the last one home pays the bill.'

MacLeod heard no more as he left the Paradise Curry House for home but, as he turned the corner of Bouverie Street, he looked back to see the entire be-kilted Running Club line up outside the door of the restaurant, chortling and hee-hawing, and the head waiter, white table napkin raised high in his hand, shout,

'Ready, **steady**, **go!**'

The napkin descended and they were off, sprinting away from the restaurant just as fast as they could manage on wobbly stomachs swollen with eight pints of lager and a curry dinner.

And they were gone, around the first corner and sprinting into the distance. In an instant, all the runners had disappeared, and were not to be seen again by the Paradise Curry House head waiter, who was left clutching the bill for the Running Club's annual dinner.

On the day after the outing, MacLeod was sitting in his office collecting together the references for his review article when the office phone rang. He reached for the phone.

'Hello? MacLeod speaking.'

It was Judith, the departmental secretary.

'It's Mr Gershon for you, MacLeod. He says that it's quite urgent. He seems cross. I can't imagine what he's got to be cross about. You better speak to him, MacLeod.'

MacLeod gulped. Mr Gershon was the medical school secretary, the man responsible for running the administrative apparatus of the school. Although Judith might not be able to imagine what Mr Gershon was cross about, MacLeod certainly could. In fact, he could easily imagine what it was that Mr Gershon was cross about. MacLeod gulped again and clenched the phone tightly as Mr Gershon, confining himself to just a few words unadorned with politeness or options, said,

'Dr MacLeod. I have just had the owner of the Paradise Curry House in my office. Would you come to my office? **Now!**'

MacLeod walked through the runnels of the hospital's basement corridors, past the porters, visitors and nurses, bustling and busy, and when he looked at the drawn faces of the patients on their trolleys and in their wheelchairs, the curse of a mortal illness was as nothing compared with the bane of Neil Gershon's wrath.

Head low, hands deep in the pockets of his white coat, MacLeod waited for the lift that would take him to the eighth floor of the tower block, the location of the medical school secretary's office. The crowd shuffled into the lift, squeezed tight to fit in yet more passengers and then bobbed up through the floors, stopping at each level to disgorge passengers, but strangely to take nobody in.

By the time MacLeod had reached the eighth floor, he was the sole occupant of the lift. Although he had done nothing personally that was wrong, he felt uncomfortable because he knew that as President of the Running Club he should have realised what the group had been up to and taken some responsibility for their actions. But he hadn't taken responsibility and his audience with Mr Gershon was the consequence of that recklessness.

MacLeod waited on an uncomfortable low leather chair in the anteroom to Mr Gershon's office, an obliquely lit anteroom occupied by two secretaries and a collection of cacti. Lining the office walls were portentous portraits of desiccated past medical school deans, posed unsmiling in their robes and mortar boards. The anteroom's single window looked on to a bare corridor where a dying neon light flashed on and off, its migrainous light inflating the anxiety felt by MacLeod as he waited for his evisceration by Mr Gershon. From time to time, one or other of the secretaries peeked over their computer screens to stare at MacLeod and it seemed to him that every time they did so, their peeking was followed by head shaking and suppressed giggling. MacLeod was made to wait for thirty-five minutes, each minute a pinprick reminder to MacLeod from Mr Gershon of the immense seriousness of the sins of the Running Club and of the enormous gravity of MacLeod's dereliction of duty.

A phone rang on one of the secretary's desks.

'Certainly, Mr Gershon. I will let him know.'

The secretary put the phone down and turned to MacLeod.
'He'll be another 30 minutes.'

'OK, I'll go for a coffee then.'

The secretary shook her head.

'No, I wouldn't do that if I were you. He's very cross.'

MacLeod nodded and turned to a contemplation of the deans. He imagined how these portraits would be viewed in another century. There the deans posed, framed in gold leaf, and swaddled in black robes bordered by ermine, velvet and silk. There they preened, cross-eyed with arrogance, staring out from their portraits, peering with immense condescension at all who would look at them, from painterly backgrounds of books and bones. MacLeod concluded that in the next century the paintings would be viewed somewhere deep in a landfill.

Meanwhile, MacLeod had been interred by Mr Gershon in a place of contrition, a contrition that was to last at least another thirty minutes. On the low glass table in front of him, there was a tidy pile of tatty medical journals. MacLeod flicked through the pile and reached for the *British Medical Journal*. As he did so, he had the distinct impression from the glare of Mr Gershon's two secretaries that it was not his place to untidy the journals, and so he deliberately scattered the magazines untidily over the table top and 'accidentally' dropped a copy of *The Lancet* on the floor.

MacLeod stretched his legs and ground his heel into the journal. He'd never managed to get an article published in *The Lancet*. The secretaries seeing this tut-tutted, and MacLeod, for the hell of it, the fizz and fuss of their irritation irritating him, stubbed his heel more firmly into the cover, with the idea that just possibly this sort of loutishness might shorten his waiting time in the anteroom. He was, of course, wrong; it only consolidated the official view of the criminal nature of the personalities of the members of the medical school Running Club.

MacLeod finished reading the *BMJ* and turned to an eight-year-old copy of *Nature*. He read on and it was time for *PNAS* and then for the *New Statesman*. The minutes dragged by and one of the secretaries left the room with a

'See you in the canteen,' to her colleague. She left without glancing at MacLeod which he took as a bad sign. MacLeod was correct – it *was* a bad sign.

MacLeod had been waiting for over an hour for his 'urgent' appointment with the medical school secretary. He considered that the point had been made about the weakness of his own position compared to the importance of the medical school secretary, and as the point had been made, surely enough time had been spent by him in the secretary's anteroom. The interconnecting telephone rang again, and it seemed that MacLeod was right – enough time had been spent teaching him his place in the medical school hierarchy. The moment had come for him to change rooms and face the man.

'Dr MacLeod, you can go in now.'

MacLeod got up and, knocking on the splendidly polished mahogany door that led into Mr Gershon's office, waited for the 'come in' that invited him to open that door.

'MacLeod!' Mr Gershon snarled, face on fire with rage, lips pursed, expression livid, fists grinding into the desk.

'What the hell were you up to, MacLeod? What the hell did you think you were doing?'

Gershon stood up and, leaning forward over his desk, brandished an evil-looking brass letter opener at MacLeod, scything the air around him with vicious lethality.

Now, this was a different Gershon to the Gershon that MacLeod was used to. MacLeod had been at school with Gershon and, at school, Gershon had been a gentle chubby fellow of amiable disposition. Gershon had been one of the few boys in the years above him who had acknowledged the presence of the younger pupils and done so not because of perversion. When MacLeod had arrived at his present hospital, Gershon had been kind enough to welcome him and wish him luck in his research post. The rant continued,

'I have had the owner of the Paradise Curry House here and he has told me what happened last night in his restaurant.'

MacLeod was perplexed by the change in Gershon's demeanour. What had happened to his mild-mannered friend?

'And furthermore, we do not expect this kind of unaccept-
able behaviour from a member of the medical school staff.'

The letter opener whooshed through the air and passed
perilously close to the upper leaves of a yucca plant on the
edge of Gershon's desk. The leaves rustled and the plant
rocked in its saucer. This was an entirely new Gershon,
aggressively truculent, incandescent and furious. Surely all
that was required was a quiet request for MacLeod to gather
together a group of the runners and apologise to the
restaurateur?

'I have to say that I am minded to take this matter up with
the Board of Studies. The students could be rusticated, you
know.'

This was surely going too far. The letter opener took
another pass through the air around Gershon's head, swooped
over the desk and decapitated the yucca plant. There was no
room in the maelstrom of Gershon's anger for an interjection
from MacLeod. Gershon, swollen with rage, engorged with
wrath, juddered over the desk, icteric with anger, bubbling
with fury. MacLeod felt that the time had come for him to try
to placate the man.

'I am very sorry, Neil. But it was only medical students
having a bit of fun.'

Gershon rustled with anger.

'Ffffffun ... ffffffun? he stuttered. 'You call that fun?'

Gershon's behaviour seemed most puzzling to MacLeod.
The school secretary leaned further forward on his desk, his
fists embedded in a pile of papers, and such was the weight of
his anger that the papers spewed across the desk and he
tipped forward slightly. He quickly regained his position but
MacLeod, distracted by the scurry of papers, was drawn
towards the books and papers on Gershon's desk. And in the
confusion of work laid out on the medical school secretary's
desk, MacLeod spotted the reason for the change in the secretary's demeanour. For there amidst the papers and files
resplendent in the most virile of red bindings lay *The Harvard
Assertiveness Bible. How You Too Can Change The Way
People View You In Eight Easy Lessons. A Multidisciplinary
Approach to Self-Assertion.*

'Ah ha …' thought MacLeod, '… so that's what he's been up to. Assertiveness training and he's trying it out on me! The medical students won't have a chance. I'll have to work to save the stupid buggers' bacon.'

'Certainly, Neil, I'm sure you're absolutely right. Really! Send 'em all up. Put them before the Board of Studies. Mind you if we do that, then they'll all be finished! They'll be out on their ears. Pity really because there are a couple of them that are potentially university gold medal material …'

MacLeod waited for the bait to be taken; he knew that possession of the university gold medal would do a lot for the medical school ratings and that the medical school ratings were really in need of a bit of a boost.

'Gold medal material you say …' The bait had been duly taken.

'Yes, Neil. Two of the students are right at the top of their classes in all of their subjects. There haven't been students like them for a long time. They're really serious candidates for the medal.'

Gershon sat down behind his desk and rested his chin on his fist.

'Hmm. Well that does put a different complexion on the matter. You'd better call them in and give them a serious warning, then after a good keelhauling take them around to that idiot at the Paradise. Make them apologise and, above all, make them pay the bloody bill. Now bugger off, MacLeod – and you'd better be right about that bloody gold medal …'

Chapter 12
In More Foreign Parts

At the completion of his postgraduate research years, MacLeod had submitted his doctoral thesis, which had earned him an appointment as consultant at a teaching hospital. He had arranged to have some holiday before taking up his post and starting the next phase of his career, which would take him to sixty-five years old, if he was lucky, when he was likely to be deaf, even more senseless and bald. The holiday consisted of a trip to New Orleans to meet an expert who had led studies in his own research field, a Nobel laureate called Andrew Schally.

Dr Schally had won his Nobel Prize in 1977 for his work on a hormone secreted by the hypothalamus called gonadotrophin releasing hormone. The hypothalamus controls ovulation and testicular function. By a complex biochemical process, Dr Schally identified the molecular structure of gonadotrophin releasing hormone. He did so by first purifying the hormone from the hypothalami of 180,000 pigs. The hypothalamus is tiny, weighing just a few grams and the dissection of this tiny organ is quite an enterprise. Dr Schally had come to an arrangement with local abattoirs to harvest hypothalami and it was a measure of his remarkable drive and focus that he had managed to complete his collection of so many pig hypothalami. The purification procedure had produced 11.4 mg of gonadotrophin releasing hormone from those 180,000 pigs.

'Quite a lot of pigs!' MacLeod had remarked to a friend.

J. Waxman, *MacLeod's Introduction to Medicine*,
DOI 10.1007/978-1-4471-4522-6_12,
© Springer-Verlag London 2014

MacLeod liked New Orleans, a city of a certain pace and beat, its climate subtropical, the muddy Mississippi tracing through its innards, tourist-hungry paddle-boat steamers at its banks. Buses threaded through the city proclaiming implausible destinations such as 'Paradise' and 'Elysian Fields'. New Orleans with its gaudily painted low-rise nineteenth-century villas, delicately decorated with iron-work tracery of balconies and verandas. New Orleans, with its thump and bash of bars and jazz clubs. Low-life New Orleans and high-life New Orleans. New Orleans with its dead buried above the water level, raised above ground in marble tombs, decayed bodies safe from rising tides, rotting flesh protected from rainstorm parades by the weight of stone. New Orleans – its seafood and its patois; New Orleans – home to the entire country's drunks, midnight cowboy migrants to the warmth of its shores; New Orleans – the city's tarts brightly lit on its main streets; New Orleans – voodoo and vaudeville.

MacLeod took a taxi to Dr Schally's laboratory, not trusting the buses to deliver him to such a prosaic destination. He thought about Dr Schally and the anecdotes about him that coloured a spectacular life. The endocrinologist was in his sixties and in his photographs looked as though he had had a hair transplant. His hair, blackened by hair dye and rigid with shining pomade, was the most noticeable feature of his appearance. His long-jawed, thin-cheeked face stared out questioning the photographer. Dr Schally had been a sports-man in his youth and had emigrated from Poland to Scotland, where he had played centre forward for Hibernian.

'There aren't many Nobel laureates who have played First Division football!' MacLeod mused, as he waited in the lobby of the Veterans Hospital for the receptionist to notify Dr Schally's secretary of his arrival.

'You can go up now,' the receptionist said, smiling with one of those American big-lipped smiles that exposes too many teeth. 'Sixth Floor, Sir. No, not that way, Sir. That's the john. The elevator's over there, honey.'

The elevator jerked upwards and juddered to a halt at the sixth floor, where the door opened to reveal Dr Schally's secretary waiting for him with a beaming smile. MacLeod shook her hand and she invited him to sit with her in her office until Dr Schally was ready to see him. They walked through a lab corridor that was strangely quiet and, in its stillness, completely unlike the messy bustle of MacLeod's own departmental laboratory.

MacLeod waited in Dr Schally's secretary's office, a modernist construction of chrome and glass, and skimmed through a science journal as the time passed until his appointment. They'd arranged for him to come up to the labs for a meeting at 4 pm. At precisely that time, the intercom on Dr Schally's secretary's desk buzzed. The secretary looked up from her correspondence folder, smiled at MacLeod and announced,

'He'll see you now. Do go in, Dr MacLeod. Have a nice day, Sir.'

MacLeod was ushered to a connecting door to Dr Schally's office. There sat the great man, protected from all comers by a formidable desk. Dr Schally's office was lined with oppressive black metal filing cabinets enigmatically labelled with white card. The windows looked out over the city and on the office walls were framed diplomas and citations, doctorates and awards, and amongst them, the grandest of all awards, a photograph of Dr Schally bowing before the King of Sweden as he accepted his Nobel Prize. Dr Schally greeted MacLeod with a cold,

'Welcome to New Orleans, Dr MacLeod,' that could not have been more unwelcoming.

MacLeod's immediate impression was of a man of great stiffness and formality. Dr Schally was dressed in a white lab coat with its collar up, white shirt, dark brown tie held in a gold tiepin, slacks and an immaculately starched lab coat. And that hair, the hair that had been such a feature of the photographs! The hair had been transplanted, grafted in great clumps into his scalp, isolated islands of evenly placed stalks of hair swimming in a sea of skin, hair greased and dyed, Brilliantined hair slicked back from his forehead and plastered back over oceans of baldness. Dr Schally extended a hand in greeting but didn't get up from his chair to shake hands. There was a great space of desk between MacLeod and Dr Schally, clear protective space without encumbrance of paper.

MacLeod sat at Dr Schally's desk, distanced from the professor by six feet of polished shiny teak. MacLeod had come to New Orleans on holiday, but on a break that combined sunbathing and fine food with a plan for future collaborative work. He hoped to agree a joint research programme with the great man. But in conversation, there was a certain reticence in Dr Schally, no wish to engage, no desire to release information that could possibly lead to the formulation of ideas for a joint project.

The conversation was leisurely, polite and focused on past discoveries. Dr Schally was guarded in conversation, confining his talk to science, restricting his discussion to work long gone. No recent laboratory findings were discussed. MacLeod understood the reason for this concentration on the past, because in science, discoveries are currency. Results have great value, and invention is the ticket for future grant income and learned publications. So, in the realm of Schally's kingdom, the air bristled with paranoia and the walled cities of intellectual property were heavily fortified. Dr Schally protected his ideas from all intruders, and did so in a manner that embodied a struggle between politeness and secrecy. He needed to preserve the work that he was doing in New Orleans from any prying mind.

Suddenly, the door to Dr Schally's office opened and the professor's wife, Dr Comaru-Schally, walked in. She wore a white lab coat, collar up, a mirror of her husband's white coat. She was small and dark haired. She was South American, co-author on all of his papers and his great love.

'This is Dr MacLeod from England; he's come to visit us.'

And Dr Comaru-Schally took MacLeod's hand, her handshake strangely formless and limp.

Further polite conversation followed and MacLeod sensed that the air of suspicion was lifting and that he was gradually being accepted as a colleague who had not come to steal their scientific ideas, as a scientist with whom they might do business. Stroking his chin, Dr Schally leaned towards Macleod and asked,

'You'd like to see the lab?'

'I'd love to see the laboratory.'

Dr Schally stood up, and MacLeod was surprised to see how tall he was. Then, followed by his wife and MacLeod, he walked out of his office into the corridor. The corridor wound around four sides of a square that enclosed the elevator shaft. In the middle of each side of the square, double doors led from the corridor into four laboratories. Windows were built into the corridor walls, so that everything that went on inside the labs could be viewed by those who passed by. Dr Schally crept along the corridor, hunched low below the glass so that he could not be seen by anyone who might have looked out from the labs. He pushed against the door of the first lab and, as it opened, sprung up to his full height. The lights were on but the lab was empty.

Dr Schally turned to MacLeod, his face expressing puzzlement. He raised his arms in amazement and shrugged.

'Extraordinary! They have gone home – so early! So, there is nothing here that I can show you! Let's move on!'

Dr Schally, bent double as he walked the corridor, a Golem-like figure, hands clasped in front of him, stooped and leery. He hesitated before the door of the second lab, and then drew himself up, nose out. He was there to drive ambition, to encourage the workers, drive the scientists on to explorations of the unknown. He was on parade to fuel discovery. And woe betide the slackers, the scientists who should be on the job; woe betide anyone who was relaxing in the lab when they ought to be hard at work.

Dr Schally turned the door handle and burst explosively into the second lab. But the second lab was empty, too; the scientists had gone home. The cell shakers reverberated, the electrophoresis apparatus sulked, the lab benches gleamed, the computers glowered, and the PCR machines pulsed. But the bottles and pipettes stood easy; there was not a researcher in the lab. Dr Schally looked crestfallen, and without an apology for the fact that there was nothing that could be shown to

MacLeod, he slammed the lab door shut and walked around the corner of the building to the third lab. Now there was no pretence at surprise. Dr Schally marched at full height, striding purposely through the corridors.

Dr Schally opened the door to the third laboratory and, to his surprise and joy, discovered a scientist at work in the lab. At a distant bench, pipette in his gloved hand, there stood quite the smallest man that MacLeod had ever seen. He was oriental and wore thick glasses. He bowed reverentially to Dr Schally, then he bowed to the professor's shadow, Dr Comaru-Schally and then he bowed again to MacLeod, but bowed not quite as reverentially as he had bowed to the professor and his wife. Dr Schally's face shone with the smile of a shark that had just enjoyed a very pleasant halibut dinner. He walked up to the scientist's bench followed by his wife and MacLeod. The scientist trembled and his pipette clattered on to the bench. Dr Schally scrutinised the gel that the scientist was in the process of loading.

'Ah, Dr Tan. So what do you have here?'

'Dr Schally, it is a gel.'

'Of course, it's a gel, Dr Tan. I know it's a gel. I have worked in science for forty years. That isn't what I meant at all. Dr Tan, my question is this. What, Dr Tan, are you doing at the moment?'

'Pipetting, Dr Schally.'

'Yes. I can see that, Dr Tan, but why are you pipetting?'

'Ah so. So that I can load the gels, Dr Schally.'

Dr Schally shook his head giving up on the idea that he might get some sense out of the man.

'Excellent. Now, Dr Tan, may I introduce you to Dr MacLeod, an esteemed visitor from the United Kingdom?'

'Yes, Dr Schally, you may introduce me to Dr MacLeod.'

'Dr MacLeod, may I introduce you to Dr Tan, who is from Taiwan and is working for us on the somatostatin protocol.'

They shook hands, and at the word 'esteemed', Dr Tan bowed again, this time bending so low that he knocked his brow on the edge of his lab worktop.

'Very good, Dr Tan. You carry on, good to see you working ... when the others ...'

Words at this point evaporated from Dr Schally's mouth. He shook his head in disbelief at the temerity of the scientists who had dared to go home before he, Dr Schally, had vacated the building. Dr Schally left Dr Tan to his pipettes and his failure to understand colloquial English and returned to his office followed by his wife and MacLeod. They sat around the professor's enormous desk and drank coffee. Dr Schally searched in his filing cabinets and then handed MacLeod reprints of some of his old publications. They were all from a previous decade. He gave him no preprints, no new information; there was nothing of excitement for MacLeod, nothing unknown to the scientific world. All that was new was kept secret for fear of the competition drawing an advantage over the home team. Dr Comaru-Schally nodded as each publication was given to MacLeod, nodded as if she was greeting an old friend.

Macleod glanced at his watch. It was 4.30 pm. Dr Schally, noticing MacLeod's action, looked at his own watch, stood up and said,

'If you aren't busy this evening, perhaps you'd like to come for supper with us?'

'That would be great,' said MacLeod. 'I'd love to. Thank you.'

It was time to go home and Dr Schally and his wife stood together by the office door wearing their lab coats, him in front of her, him with his back to her, her, his little shadow. The professor shifted from side to side, swaying gently as he patted his various pockets checking for keys and wallets and pens and whatever else he needed to check for and Dr Comaru-Schally's movements echoed those of her husband's. It was a pas de deux of unusual character. Then, satisfied that all was in place in the pockets of his life, Dr Schally checked all of the locks of all of the filing cabinets, shuffled through the tidy pile of uncrumpled papers on his desk, grabbed a briefcase, emptied the pile of papers into his briefcase, and stepped from the office, Dr Comaru-Schally trailing him and MacLeod following close behind.

Into the elevator and down to the ground floor of the lab block, the three of them went in silence. In the context of a world where lab coats are usually left in laboratories for fear of plague and contagion, unusually the two Doctor Schally's had remained in their white coats as they descended in the elevator and walked through the foyer. They strode on in their pristine, gleaming, crisply starched lab coats, their scary white coats, white coats that denoted what the Schally's thought of as important in their world. Their walk was conjoined, linked in pace and stride. In the company of the Schally's in their bright white coats, collars up, MacLeod, white coat-less, was a lunatic on parole from the asylum, escorted by two nurses on a day outing.

The Schally's walked through the car park to an elderly, standard issue American car with muted fins and a long bonnet. Dr Schally sat in the driver's seat, checking his wing mirrors, checking his rear-view mirror, adjusting the seat, adjusting his coat, inspecting his image in the rear-view mirror, adjusting the position of his seat again, and then with a jerk that brought back to Macleod memories of Professor Katz, they were off and out of the car park, and pushed into the traffic with an entire disregard for lane priorities. The rush-hour traffic was dense but the traffic flowed, and windows up, air conditioning on, the Schally's coasted forward and drifted onwards. Dr Schally, disregarding his responsibility to the other drivers, hands stiff on the wheel, turned to MacLeod. He nodded and said,

'First, we are going home to change.'

'Great!' said MacLeod.

'Do you swim, MacLeod?' MacLeod noted that he had been addressed with familiarity and friendship, his formal title dropped – he had been promoted!

They had been driving for 100 yards with Dr Schally looking backwards into the interior of the car. Remarkably, the car had not strayed from its lane. Macleod stared ahead with terror. A bend in the road approached.

'Turn around you, bastard!' MacLeod prayed that his chauffeur would turn to look where he was going, but Dr Schally did not turn around. No! Dr Schally stared meaningfully at MacLeod, his arm draped over the back of his seat, and said,

'We have a pool, you know.'

Then to MacLeod's great relief, Dr Schally turned just in time and steered the car around a ferocious bend.

The car had proceeded on its stately way through the suburbs of New Orleans. Dr Schally seemed to enjoy the steering in particular and made a great thing of ushering the steering wheel through his hands with enormous deliberation. The suburban roads were wide and lined with deep lawns that led up to clapboard houses. Suddenly the professor jerked the steering wheel to the right and clipping the curb, bumped across a lawn and onto a short driveway, where the car stalled in front of the doors of his garage. Dr Schally took the key from the ignition, looked around the front garden with huge suspicion, pushed open the car door and swung his long legs out and onto the pathway that led to his front door. Dr Comaru-Schally followed her husband, her pace and posture again mirroring her husband as he marched across crisp gravel to a very small bungalow with an overwhelmingly fortified front door, bulked up with a lattice of steel grills and draped with wrought-iron chains and heavy padlocks.

'So, there are no problems with burglars here? Looks like a peaceful neighbourhood, Dr Schally?' MacLeod commented ironically. But the professor did not 'do' irony.

'The neighbourhood is very safe. That's why we live here. But nonetheless, MacLeod, we do have to be careful.'

Dr Schally pulled a chain of keys from his pocket and opened the padlocks. He released the chains from the steel grill and, opening his front door, beamed at his esteemed colleague from the United Kingdom.

'Come in, come in, MacLeod. Sit down, make yourself at home. My wife will make you a drink. What would you like?'

MacLeod sat down on a brown leather sofa, which occupied most of the front room of the house. On the walls there were aerial photographs of Rio and an enormous rectangular digital clock. The room was dominated by this clock which screamed out the time in an alarmingly bright red LED display. The digital time throbbed on and then off, on and then off; it was quite the scariest clock MacLeod had ever seen.

MacLeod and Dr Schally were given glasses of orange juice by Dr Comaru-Schally and Professor Schally, slapping his glass on to the coffee table, stood up and announced,

'I have to go and change now.'

Professor Schally nodded at MacLeod and left the room to emerge through a different door in swimming briefs that were alarmingly tight.

'I must do my lengths.'

The Noble laureate peered out into the garden with caution.

'Who knows what he thinks is out there,' thought MacLeod.

Although it was bright daytime, the laureate switched on the garden lights. Great floodlights burst on to the flowerbeds and Dr Schally looked outside with enormous suspicion. He unbolted and slid open the French windows that led to the garden. His hand on the window frame, so as to close it on any marauder, he poked his head cautiously into the garden. He withdrew into the room and waited a few seconds for gangs of criminals to appear. Then, with not a burglar, axe murderer, rapist or masked assassin in view, the professor ventured carefully into the garden and stepped towards the pool.

A moment later MacLeod heard Dr Schally mumbling and grumbling as he walked around the pool, complaining about a gardener who had not paid sufficient attention to the cleaning of the pool. It was clear from the loud complaints that Dr Schally suspected the gardener had used the pool to swim when he should have been working. The professor curled his toes around the edge of the pool, stretched, and raised his arms above his head. He tipped forward. Suddenly there was a great and inelegant splash as Dr Schally bellyflopped into the pool.

Dr Comaru-Schally had been at the French windows watching her husband dive in and with that splash she turned her attention to her guest. She sat down on the couch next to MacLeod and patted the cushion between them with her hand. She moved uncomfortably close to MacLeod.

'I am from Brazil,' she said and, looking at him meaningfully, she winked.

'Really?' said MacLeod, sweating a little and wondering what was coming next.

'Yes, from Rio, actually. You know Rio?'

'Can't say that I do.'

Dr Comaru-Schally squeezed closer to MacLeod.

'In Rio, we have the carnival. You've heard about the carnival, no? I have a magazine from the carnival. You'd like to look, no?'

'Thank you.'

MacLeod took the magazine from Dr Comaru-Schally and opened it to a parade of very scantily clad women, views of Rio that he felt he should not be sharing with a married woman tightly squeezed next to him on the sofa. At that point, just when the heat seemed too much for MacLeod to bear, Professor Schally came bursting in from the garden dripping water onto the shag pile. His chest hair was matted from his exertion but his hair transplant was an immaculate rug that had held its form and colour.

'Ana Maria!' he exclaimed, and MacLeod was reminded of a certain Beatrix Potter character calling for provisions.

'We should take MacLeod to supper, Ana Maria.'

Within a few minutes, Professor Schally was dry and the little group were off in the car venturing through the streets to the restaurant. Dr Comaru-Schally had not, MacLeod noticed, taken off her white coat and Dr Schally had put his white coat back on. It was around 5.30 pm, a trifle early for supper in Blighty.

'But in foreign parts,' thought MacLeod, 'do as the foreign parts do.' MacLeod was always ready to eat.

The car cruised at 15 mph, its progress majestic, doors locked against the vicissitudes of violence. They arrived at the parade of shops where the restaurant was located and parked the car in a broad forecourt. It wasn't a grand place. Far from grand, it was the New Orleans equivalent of a fish and chip shop. But instead of rock and chips, the deep fry offered 'Oysters Rockefeller'. The proprietor greeted the group with deference. Professor Schally introduced his guest to him. The proprietor wiped his fists on a dish cloth and offered MacLeod his hand. He leaned over a gleaming glass counter and said,

'Welcome to New Orleans, Sir. I hear you hail from England. And how is the Queen?' This said with considerable politeness, a serious enquiry. And the answer – well it had to be,

'Her Majesty is very well, thank you.'

The Oysters Rockefeller were served to MacLeod on a paper plate with chips. In later years, he looked up the recipe but in the cookbooks the recipe for Oysters Rockefeller didn't correspond to what he'd been served that night. The New Orleans' chip shop produced deep-fried oysters wrapped in spinach. The three of them stood eating these oysters while the chip-shop proprietor watched them from behind the counter, doffing his head in deference to Professor Schally's every word, dazed and deeply reverential of his fame. The two scientists ate in their lab coats. The restaurant was icy cool, the air conditioning was full on. And then suddenly it was 6 pm; good night time – and time, indeed, for a taxi ride back to his hotel.

MacLeod returned home from his American 'holiday' to begin his life sentence, a consultancy at a famous London teaching hospital. At the end of the first couple of years of his prison term, MacLeod started a fundraising appeal for a new ward block. This appeal aimed to replace a ghastly Victorian workhouse-style hospital with a modern building. The old building looked like a prison. It had an antique roof, which had no interesting patina, and let in the rain. The windows were barred and the walls were graced with fungus which crept decorously through peeling plasterwork. Although some of the patients liked the patterns made by the fungus, none of them was that keen on the raindrops that dripped on their beds.

The original spark for the appeal had been lit during a conversation that MacLeod had had with one of the patients. The man was waiting on a steel trolley for a porter to take him to the X-ray department, in a corridor that whistled with wind. The bristling breeze ruffled the patient's bed linen, and exposed his toes. MacLeod stopped to chat. The patient looked up at MacLeod from his trolley and said,

'I really don't understand how you can work in this environment! You know, Doctor, it's bad enough that we patients suffer in these conditions. But you, Doctor, you have to spend your whole working life here!'

So the fundraising campaign followed and efforts were made to raise money for a modern hospital building. The campaign was pump-primed by a self-effacing philanthropist who donated £1 million and didn't expect a knighthood for his anonymous gift. As appeals went, the appeal went well and MacLeod soon had enough money to employ slick fundraising executives and organise fundraising dinners, and the occasional fundraising lunch.

One of the lunches was held at the House of Commons, and it was there that MacLeod met two more Nobel laureates, Max Perutz and Fred Sanger. Max was another of Hitler's gifts: born in Austria, a gifted writer, his accent heavily Germanic. Max had won the Nobel Prize in 1962 for establishing the crystal structure of haemoglobin. Max was full of fun and he was sitting next to Fred, who was shy and so overcome with shyness that he was virtually mute unless directly questioned. Fred had won two Nobel prizes, which made him rather exceptional. The first was awarded in 1958 for working out the structure of insulin and the second in 1980 for establishing a technique for sequencing the structure of DNA. His endeavours were carried out quietly and without fuss. He had no huge research team, but just got on with it, working without a retinue, busy, but busy quietly, without fuss and with just a single technician at his side.

MacLeod walked through the grand gothic entrance to the Commons, ornate and pointy, and stomped across the Pugin pavement. The corridor walls were bordered with dark oak and papered with grand gilt-framed paintings. He strolled into the central lobby, a crossroads of four concourses. There, the MPs and their assistants scurried to meetings, sweeping through the corridors, making turbulence with their sheaves of papers and loud voices. From the crossroads, Macleod was directed to a huge dining area where tables had been laid with white cloths and arrayed with glistening silver. There were wine bottles on the tables, and the numbers of the great and the good in attendance that afternoon seemed to be less than the numbers of wine bottles set on the tables. The crowd laughed and joked and seemed at home in what was to MacLeod a very unfamiliar and un-homely environment. The maître d' called for attention, places were found by the shuffling crowd, grace was said, and a polite speech was delivered by Lord Thisandthat welcoming all of the guests and reminding them of the nobility of the fundraising cause which was the pivotal point of the proceedings.

MacLeod, sitting at the same table as Perutz and Sanger, with a certain nervousness watched the lunch being served and eaten. That nervousness had at its core his concern that the guest of honour had not as yet turned up. This guest of honour was the host of a certain radio show that finished at midday – and midday was long passed. It was dessert time, and still there was no sign of the guest of honour.

'Ah, there he is …'

And the buzz of recognition that greeted the arrival of the famous man was palpable. Terry Logan glided into the Commons dining room, smiling, shaking hands with friends, waving at the crowd, working the room. He was master of bonhomie, hospitality's radiator. His presence at the function added an additional 50 % to the donations that would be put in the box that afternoon. Logan stepped up to the microphone offered him by the master of ceremonies and delivered an encomium focusing on the nobility of the cause, the need to help those in need, and the general excellence of the excellent hospital for which the excellent Appeal was aspiring to build a new unit. At the end of his speech, Logan drew his audience's attention to the brown envelopes that were positioned under their plates and asked all present to make a significant donation. It was a great speech, and all the envelopes were filled.

Logan was guided from his podium to a place of honour in the audience, opposite Perutz and Sanger. His glossy black toupee was squew-whiff and his cheeks were red. As he sat down, he whispered to the master of ceremonies:

'A double vodka tonic, please. Go easy on the tonic and hard on the vodka. You'll know what I mean, friend. A thousand blessings on your house. Thanks very much.'

Logan turned to his meal which had been kept warm for him, and tucked in, white linen napkin thrust into his collar. His new lifelong best friend, a waiter returned with his drink.

'Ah, that's a relief. I'm as dry as the Sahara.' He knocked back the vodka. 'There's mother's milk for you. Thank goodness. Well done, that man. Your reward will be in heaven. Make that another large one would you, friend?'

Logan twinkled with bonhomie and looked visibly relieved as the vodka coursed through his system and anaesthetised his tremulous parts. Feeling a little more relaxed, Logan ate on and then put down his knife and fork, and patted at his lips with his napkin. Unbeknown to him, Logan had been the subject of scrutiny during his meal. Max Perutz had been staring at him with more than a casual curiosity as he had drunk his vodka and eaten his lunch. But now it was coffee time, and all was easy at the top of the top table.

Max said,

'Very good of you to come to help with the fundraising cause, Mr Logan. Thank you!'

'My pleasure! Think nothing of it at all, friend.'

Fred Sanger had also been staring at Logan as he ate and drank. Conscious of the laureate's gaze, Logan glanced at his neighbour's place card and for conversation asked,

'So you are Fred, and *what* do you do Fred, for a living?'

'Well, Mr Logan ...' Dr Sanger stuttered, 'I'm a s s s s scientist.'

'Ah, so you're a scientist? Jolly good show. Boiling, bubbling test tubes and all that hocus pocus. Is that it? And tell me, Fred do you have any fluorescent rats?'

'Well, Mr Logan. Test tubes, yes, bbbbut not exactly fluorescent rats ...'

'I see now, Fred, so there are test tubes. That's a relief, I'm sure, but there aren't rats? And that's a shame, but not a shame for the rats who are clearly well out of it. How about the white coats, Fred? I do hope there are white coats. And great cauldrons of hissing blue fluid? Please tell me that there are cauldrons in the lab.'

'Not quite, Mr Logan. Lab coats, yes, bbbbut not exactly cauldrons. We do have retorts and there are Bunsen burners still.'

'Ah! Bunsen burners, takes me right back to my school-days. Garçon, Garçon, another of these, would you mind? Just to steady the nerves. Thank you, there's a good man.'

Logan leaned forward and his elbow missed the edge of the table. His toupee slipped as he slipped, but he was oblivious to everything, focusing on teasing Fred Sanger. Max Perutz listened quietly as his friend was tormented.

'Now, Fred, have you heard my show on the radio?'

'I am terribly sorry, bbbbut I don't really listen much to the radio. I do try to concentrate on my work in the daytime.'

'Oh well, can't say you've missed much. So, what have you discovered in your work?'

'Oh, nnnnothing much.'

'Can't say that I've discovered much in mine either, old chap!' and Logan roared with laughter.

Max Perutz leaned into the conversation watching his friend, listening intently. Logan continued,

'But you science chappies, you're usually up to something. I know you lot! You scientist types! Off you go, making some great discovery before breakfast. What do you lot get up to?'

'Nnnnnothing really, Mr Logan ...'

At this point, Max Perutz could stand it no longer.

'So, tell him about ze Nobel Prize, Fred ...'

'You've won a Nobel Prize?' Logan turned to Dr Sanger and looked at him with interest.

'Wwwwell actually ...' Dr Sanger squirmed with embarrassment. And as he squirmed, Max laughed and, chuckling, mumbled in a loud voice,

'So Fred, so tell him about ze two Nobel Prizes. Nein?'

'Wwwwell, actually ...'

And MacLeod smiled and thought,

'Not much that can beat that.'

Chapter 13
The Final Examinations

In their final qualifying exams, students have to prove their competence to their examiners and examiners have to prove their intellectual superiority to their fellow examiners. In these moments of anxiety and tension, there are hours of theatre. The stress of the exam setting leads the students to make the most incredible gaffes, whilst the competitiveness of the examiners produces displays of the most monstrous pomposity.

The prospect of toasting students alive is greeted with joy by examiners because of the chance of a break in the march of humdrum routine. MacLeod enjoyed being an examiner, and he aimed to pass as many medical students as he possibly could. He considered that it was part of his mission to save the Government the enormous expense of a wasted medical school education, if a student was failed. And, besides, he felt sorry for the poor buggers.

MacLeod returned to Barts to examine medical students for their finals. He remembered his own time in research at the hospital with great fondness. Walking through the medieval arch that led into the main hospital square, MacLeod felt as though the stones of the buildings had memories, and seeing him pass, the great grey building blocks seemed to whisper, 'It's him again; he's here again, here again.' And although the thought was clearly mad, MacLeod liked the idea that the buildings had a commentary for all who passed within their walls.

J. Waxman, *MacLeod's Introduction to Medicine*,
DOI 10.1007/978-1-4471-4522-6_13,
© Springer-Verlag London 2014

Walking into the main square, MacLeod was confronted with a sign that pointed the way to the MB examinations and was soon chatting with old friends and competing for the Jammy Dodgers over coffee. It seemed to him as though no time had passed at all. They knew each other well; most had been students together. Looking at the group of men sitting around the coffee table in the senior common room, MacLeod considered that everyone looked pretty much the same as they had when they were students, except for the greying hair and the flab. They were all recognisable extensions of the callow youths that they had been.

It appeared to MacLeod that the passing of the years had been as nothing. With a smile, he reflected that they could have been transported forward in time from a student flat all those years ago and there would have been not the slightest bump in the space–time continuum to mark the migration. He wondered if the future would have been predictable then, and looking around at the group of men he felt that it could have been. They'd all been bright students from middle-class families and here they were, bright-enough doctors continuing the ways of their families.

Coffee time passed with talk of this and that, until a very nervy invigilator clutching a clipboard came to usher the examiners down the long grey corridors to the outpatient's department. Part of outpatient's had been sealed off for the examinations and a maelstrom of fuss massed over the area. Several of the more senior junior doctors had been roped in to help with the organisation of the exams, and they stood behind the outpatient's clerks' desk, replete with their clipboards, looking efficient and directing the students and the examiners to their stations.

MacLeod had been briefed on his role as an examiner over coffee. The head examiner had explained that they would be examining medical students over 'short' or 'long' cases. The examiners were paired up, each pair taking turns with alternate students either to ask questions or to mark the examination candidate. MacLeod and his partner were delegated to take medical students through short cases. The patients were

volunteers and had physical troubles that were relatively
stable. Most had volunteered out of a sense of duty to mankind, a sense of duty that also involved a cash reward. Most
had performed their duty, time and time again. They were old
lags, used to the madness that seemed to erupt from the students at exam time.

The patients had been housed in individual clinic rooms or
'stations'. At each of these stations, examiners grilled the students, as they examined these hands and that spleen, that
cardiac murmur and this liver. The students were expected to
make spot diagnoses, discuss the causes of the abnormalities
that they'd found, and consider treatment and prognosis. It
was standard stuff, basic medicine. All that was required of
the student was a modicum of sense, a decent manner, gentle-
ness with the patient, and a diagnosis somewhere in the right
planetary system. The student would be passed even without
a correct diagnosis, as long as he went about things in the
right way, arranging the patient decorously as he exposed
their bellies or breasts, showing politeness as he opened and
lifted shirts and nightdresses, asking whether the patient
minded if they listened to their hearts, enquiring whether the
patient would be comfortable if they were lain flat so he
could palpate an abdominal organ.

MacLeod's fellow examiner, his partner for the morning,
was not someone that he'd met before. The man was some-
what austere, his suit double-breasted and chalk striped. He
was bald, bow tied, and pompous, and he walked along the
corridors with gait of an ostrich on an outing to the seaside.
He'd introduced himself to MacLeod as Dr Jones, tipping
forward on his toes to offer him a handshake. MacLeod was
puzzled to meet a man with 'doctor' as a first name. The
handshake was damp, his manner ingratiating. He was not
MacLeod's sort of man.

MacLeod and Jones were led along the corridor by one of
the junior doctors to a series of rooms which each had a sheet
of paper Sellotaped to their door. On the paper was a number
and the number encoded the diagnosis of the patient within,
a diagnosis written on the clipboard handed to MacLeod.

'Right,' said the junior doctor, 'I'll bring the candidate along in a moment. You'll have them with you for thirty minutes. You need to mark them out of ten.'

'Ah,' said Dr Jones, 'mark them for dress sense?'

'I don't think so, Sir!' chirruped the junior doctor.

MacLeod chuckled and thought,

'He's not that bad after all. I misjudged the bugger.'

MacLeod and Jones knocked on the door of their allotted cubicle and introduced themselves to the patient within. The patient seemed like a hermit in a cell looking up from her wheelchair to the strangers at the door. Dr Jones thanked her for giving her time so generously and MacLeod mentioned that they, the examiners, weren't really as cruel as they might appear to be and would do their best to pass all the candidates.

'Your first candidate, gentlemen.'

The junior doctor assisting in the exams ushered a volatile nervous woman into the room. Her teeth were chattering, she was dressed in black, her skirt was short but not too short, hair tied tight back in a neat bun, glasses tipped at the end of a very pretty nose. It was the prettiest nose of the morning and gave MacLeod hope for the day.

'Candidate Number 16.'

'Thanks.'

Dr Jones led the way and MacLeod muttered to the woman,

'Don't worry; I'm sure you'll be fine,' which seemed to set those teeth into a fierce waltz. She drew her hand to her neck and clutched at her pearls.

'This is the first candidate,' said Dr Jones introducing the student to the patient.

The patient, cosy in her powder-blue dressing gown, her hair nicely permed in ringlets of tight purple curls, looked up from her wheelchair and said,

'Hello, dear. I s'pect you'll want to look at my hands won't you, love? They all want to look at my hands. Don't know why they want to keep staring at them, they look so awful what with the artheritus.'

There was palpable relief on the medical student's face, as she heard the patient give away her diagnosis. But then MacLeod observed the relief turn to agitation as the thought 'what type of arthritis?' swept like a thousand storms through the candidate's mind. She twisted at her pearls and stared gloomily at the patient.

'Would you like to exam this lady's hands?' asked Dr Jones.

'Yes.'

'The perfect answer,' thought MacLeod. 'She's scored 100 % so far. The woman is clearly going to have a star-studded medical career.'

The medical student asked the patient's permission to examine her hands and taking her right hand in her own left hand stared at it with great intensity. The hand was gnarled and deformed, twisted by years of a destructive arthritis that had warped the joints. The student sweated and shook. Bright rivulets of sweat drew silver lines on her forehead and trickled along the bridge of her nose. The student looked up to the ceiling seeking the diagnosis in the depths of a light bulb, the residence of the patron saint of medical students. But Bacchus had not even been beatified, yet alone canonised, and given his history, it would have been unlikely that he would have been so assiduous in his studies that he would have been able to provide a diagnosis for the student.

There were no messages coming in from above and the medical student was floundering. The patient's hand was turned over and then over again in the medical student's hands. She enclosed the patient's hands in her own and then, uncurling the patient's fingers, she ran her thumb over the patient's palm. The student stooped low over the hand and peered at it over the frame of her glasses. She then inspected the patient's nails.

'She must be checking for clubbing,' MacLeod thought, looking for clubbing of the fingers. There was no clubbing, and there was no cyanotic change either. The nails were perfectly unremarkable.

The student started to shake and her nervousness and fear was transmitted to the patient whose arm began to ricochet up and down. The level of stress in the little cubicle was coruscating: fear stalked the bedclothes, terror screamed from the wheelchair, anxiety flapped the bed sheets.

A knowing look suddenly creased the student's face. Her eyelids narrowed and her nostrils flared.

'It's arthritis!' she pronounced.

MacLeod and Jones nodded in agreement.

'It is indeed arthritis,' said Dr Jones.

The student shook with relief.

'Excellent!' Dr Jones continued. 'And could you kindly tell us what form of arthritis our friend has?'

'Yes, Sir.'

'Good. So, what form of arthritis?'

'Ah – it's bad arthritis.'

'Excellent. Well done.'

MacLeod and Jones nodded their encouragement at the poor student.

'And would you kindly examine this lady's pulse?'

The student sighed with great relief and turned the patient's hand upwards and clasping her wrist attempted to locate the radial pulse. The patient smiled benignly at the student and said,

'It's the other side of the wrist, dear, you'll be wanting.'

The student gulped, tipped her spectacles up along the bridge of her nose and clenched her teeth.

'Thank you.'

MacLeod and Jones watched with interest as the medical student, baffled by the mysteries of the pulse, made efforts to locate it.

'I've found it!'

'Very good, very good indeed. And is there anything that you can tell us about the nature of the pulse?'

'It is present, Sir.'

Dr Jones seemed unable to contain himself.

'I think that's generally a very good sign in a patient,' he mumbled, and then covered his mouth so that the laughter within was suppressed.

'… and the rhythm?'

'Yes. It is in rhythm, Sir.'

'Very good, very good indeed. I think we'd better move on now to the heart. Would you kindly examine the heart?"

The medical student had been brought back from the brink of tears by the kindness of the examiners and, with some confidence, helped the patient onto the bed and primping the pillows asked her if she was comfortable.

'Yes, thank you dear. As long as you don't ask me to lie flat, I'll be just fine.'

The medical student stood back to contemplate her patient. Then, arranging the bedclothes neatly over the woman, she asked,

'Would you mind if I lift your nightie up, so that I can listen to your heart?'

'Of course, dear. Lost all my modesty a long time ago. It's what happens when you have a heart murmur. It's my mitral stenosis, they say.'

The medical student smirked. She knew now what she would expect to find.

MacLeod considered that the patient's revelation would probably not help the medical student come to a diagnosis.

Dr Jones and Dr MacLeod stood side by side watching the medical student as she attempted to examine the patient's heart. They noticed her warm the bell of her stethoscope with her hand before she placed the stethoscope on the patient's chest. That got the student points because it meant that she had sensitivity and concern for the patient's comfort. The student continued to do well. They were both delighted that the medical student had managed to identify that the patient's heart was on the left side of her chest. They'd not been convinced that she would even manage to find the heart given the standard of her examination of the patient's hands and pulse.

The patient lay back on the pillows, her breasts exposed. The medical student, stethoscope in her ears, braced herself to listen to the woman's heart. The patient had very large breasts. The student lifted up the left breast with her left hand and shuffled the bell of the stethoscope across the left side of the woman's chest. She inched the bell towards the woman's armpit. A puzzled look appeared on the student's face and she bent closer to the woman, as if by doing so, she would be able to hear the heart sounds more clearly. The student hunched lower and then lower, until her left cheek nestled against the patient's breast, the patient's nipple nuzzling her ear. She stooped over the woman, and her mouth dropped open. She tilted her head in concentration and her eyelids narrowed. And then a triumphant smile creased her face.

'I can hear it!' she exclaimed. 'Yes it's there, it's a murmur, and I can definitely hear it. Sounds like a train, it's amazing.'

The examiners were not convinced.

'It's a train is it? Virgin or Great Western?' MacLeod was tempted to enquire. But the situation was rescued from farce by Dr Jones who enquired decorously,

'Could you tell us a little more?'

MacLeod thought that they might be pushing their luck to expect any more detail from the candidate, but he was wrong. There was more to come:

'Yes, it's just like one of those old steam trains rushing out of a station.'

'Excellent!' remarked Dr Jones. 'Just like a steam train, indeed.'

'Now, can you help us, please, with this lady's eyes? I'd like you to examine the retina and give us a diagnosis. We'd like you to tell us what you think is wrong.'

The student trembled and reached for the arm of the patient's wheelchair for support.

Dr Jones passed an ophthalmoscope to the student. She shook and shivered; her face blanched. MacLeod thought that she might faint. But no, she gathered strength, took the ophthalmoscope from Dr Jones, and smiled politely at him.

'Thank you,' she said, struggling to switch on the machine.

The student peered at the ophthalmoscope. She twisted it in her hand trying to work out how to switch it on. She turned it upside down looking for a hidden switch. And then, staring again at the ceiling for inspiration, pursed her lips and wrestled with the ophthalmoscope, twisting the head of the machine on its body. Dr Jones took it from her and switched it on.

The student tensed and turning to the patient waved the ophthalmoscope in the air. Bright light flickered around the room and momentarily blinded the examiners who ducked to avoid the dancing light beam. The student asked the patient to look up at the ceiling and leaning over her prepared to examine her eyes.

'Please could you keep your eyes wide open and fix them on a point on the ceiling. Thanks. Yes, that point there.' And the student waved vaguely at a point over in the corner of the cubicle.

MacLeod and Jones looked with interest at the proceedings. The patient wallowed in the bed; her breasts remained exposed. She gazed up at the ceiling.

'Will that do you, love?'

'Yes, thank you.'

The student's arm flailed around in an arc and the ophthalmoscope traced a circuit of light on the walls of the cubicle. The student drew the ophthalmoscope towards her face as she prepared to examine the patient's retina. She placed her left hand on the patient's chest to steady herself, and stooped down to peer in the woman's eye. A whisk of hair escaped from the clasp of her hair clip and fluttered over the patient's face.

MacLeod and Jones stared with some amazement as the student's hand, ophthalmoscope tightly clenched, arched closer, and closer, and closer to the student's face. MacLeod and Jones stared because the light of the ophthalmoscope marched onto the student's face instead of shining into the patient's eyes. The student was pointing the ophthalmoscope in the wrong direction! The student, dazzled by the ophthalmoscope's beam, leaned into the patient's face looking for clues. The ophthalmoscope shook. MacLeod and Jones were transfixed.

'What is she doing?'

Light on, ophthalmoscope pointing in quite the wrong direction, the student frantically stared into the instrument's light source, blinded by the brightness of the beam.

MacLeod and Jones stared speechlessly at the scene, breathless with incredulity.

'What is she doing?' they thought in unison.

And then from the depths of the patient's face came the stuttering voice of the medical student,

'It's awfully bbbbright.'

The student twisted the ophthalmoscope in her hand. Bright light splashed for a moment onto her face and then spread onto her jacket. She looked up, quite dazzled, and said,

'It's awfully bright in there.'

Jones had mercy, took the ophthalmoscope from the student and switched it off.

'That's quite right. It is very bright. But well done. An excellent examination of the retina. Time's up. That'll be all, thank you. You've done very well, very well indeed.'

The medical student straightened up, took a moment to adjust to the normal light of the room and smiled at the examiners.

'Yes, thank you. Thank you very much,' echoed MacLeod. 'That'll be all for the short cases. If you'd like to go outside now, you'll be taken to the long case by the invigilators. Thanks again. That was very good.'

The medical student shuffled out of the room, feeling for the walls, half blinded, shivering and shaking, close to tears. The door closed and MacLeod turned to Jones.

'What do you think?'

'She was frightful.'

'Are we going to fail her?'

'No, we can't do that. It's her third attempt at finals. She's not allowed another chance. If we fail her, she won't ever become a doctor. That's a terrible waste of taxpayers' money.'

'But what about her future patients? She's useless. People are bound to die if she's allowed to practise medicine.'

'Don't worry, MacLeod, she'll be supervised by registrars during her houseman years and so she won't be able to do any damage to anyone. Now listen, old boy; she's pretty! She'll be snapped up! She'll marry and have kids. She'll leave medicine after her house jobs and then come back to work in middle age after re-training. I'll bet that she will eventually go into general practice where she'll be nice to people and carry out the occasional cervical smear. No potential for harm there!'

'Oh well, if you say so. By the way, our next patient – I can't believe that he's agreed to let the students carry out a pelvic exam.'

'Yes, nice chap; very good of him. You're right though, MacLeod; I wouldn't want a platoon of medical students up my jacksie.'

In a room just off the main corridor, MacLeod and Jones had coffee and ate more Jammy Dodgers. And then it was,

'Time for the next candidate. Can't be worse than that girl.'

'Fancy a bet? Five pounds? Two to one odds?'

Hooting with laughter, they returned to the invigilator's desk and were directed to another cubicle. They introduced themselves to the patient, a rather fey young man who, it turned out, was an actor, paid to participate in the examinations. He was dressed in red pyjamas and a plaid dressing gown. His hair was lank brown and parted on the right, swooping down over his face in a limp bob. He was apparently 'resting' and very happy to be helping the next generation of doctors in any way that he could. MacLeod wondered about the number of ways that he might help.

It was MacLeod's turn to ask questions and Jones's turn to observe the assessment. There was a knock on the door and Candidate 112 entered the room. They knew he was Candidate 112 because a scruffy square of paper pinned to his jumper announced that he was Candidate 112. Otherwise, they would have had difficulty knowing that he was a medical student. His shoes were scuffed and he was unshaven. Shampoo may have been in contact with his scalp sometime in the previous century, but there was a possibility that it had not. MacLeod would not have wanted to be served in a garage by Candidate 112, let alone have him carry out any intimate assessment of his person. And yet there was something endearing about the boy. Maybe it was that crooked smile and the blue eyes, maybe it was the skew-whiff tie that rolled uncomfortably from under a bedraggled collar and meandered over an eggy jumper?

The boy was made to feel at ease by MacLeod who uttered a series of platitudes that he could hardly believe that he was saying. His comments were about the weather and clinical training, the fact that the finals exams were not really serious and that he shouldn't worry at all because the people who did badly in their finals often made the greatest success of their lives. The boy grinned and did not seem to have been made more anxious by MacLeod's inept attempts to make him feel more relaxed.

'Now,' said MacLeod, 'you know that we have to make a practical assessment of your clinical skills and at this point require that you carry out a rectal examination.'

MacLeod's explanation was interrupted by a fit of coughing from Dr Jones. MacLeod wondered about that coughing, and then stopped wondering and focused on his role as an examiner.

'Yes …' he continued, '…a rectal examination.'

The aim of the assessment was to ensure that students were able to carry out clinical examinations on qualification.

The boy, MacLeod noticed, was doing well. He'd arranged the actor decorously on his side, head on a pillow, curled up in the foetal position, exposing the minimal amount of flesh necessary. He'd prepared the 'patient' for the rectal examination by telling him exactly what it was that he was going to do to him in the next few moments.

'So far, so good,' thought MacLeod.

'I am just going to put on a glove,' said the boy continuing his explanation to the patient.

'That's OK,' said the patient, from the depths of the pillow, sounding rather disappointed about the introduction of the glove.

'And then I'm just going to put a little jelly on the glove …'

'Yes,' said the actor authoritatively, knowing all about the jelly.

'… and put the gloved finger up your tail end and have a good feel around.'

MacLeod nodded encouragingly at the student. The exam candidate was doing well. He'd put the 'patient' at his ease, explained cogently what he was about to do and was behaving in an entirely professional manner.

'Excellent! Full marks so far. But then ...' thought MacLeod, 'it's not me who's doing the marking, is it? Jones is the one with the marks, it's Jones the Mark, boyo.'

'Would you like to tell us of your findings, please? Tell us what you're doing as you're doing it. Give us a commentary.'

The student placed his left hand on the patient's hip and, turning to face his examiners, explained what he was doing.

'I am making sure that the patient is comfortable and in a proper position for the procedure.'

The student turned to the patient.

'Could you bring your knees up a little more tightly to your chest please? That's it! Right up! Maybe put your arms around your knees. Great! That's really great. Thank you. Thanks!'

Left hand resting on the patient's left hip, back bent, gloved right hand approaching the patient's backside, the student continued with his monologue, explaining to his examiners precisely what he was doing. The student looked up at MacLeod, concentrating on the reaction of his examiner to his statements, pleased that he seemed to be getting things right, as judged by the nods of encouragement that accompanied his explanations.

As the gloved hand approached the patient's derrière, a glob of lubricant jelly dripped from the student's outstretched index finger and splattered on to the floor, making an unpleasant thwack.

'I am going to make an assessment of anal tone.'

The gloved hand continued on its route to anal tone and the pouting bottom of the patient awaited the assessment.

The student continued to look up at MacLeod, left hand on patient's hip, tie dangling. Focusing on his commentary and distracted by the thwack, the student failed to notice that his dangling tie intersected the approach of his glove. MacLeod noticed, but too late as the finger pushed into the tie and the tie and the finger pushed together into the patient's bum. The inexorable progress of the tie and the finger pulled the student downwards.

A quizzical look crossed the student's face from between the patient's cheeks. And the quizzical look became a look of horror as the student realised what he'd done. Then, with great presence of mind, the student said …

'Scissors please.'

And scrabbling through the drawers of the instrument trolley placed beside the bed, MacLeod found a surgical pack and opening it, tipped out scissors and handed them to the student. The student, transfixed by his tie, looked up from between the patient's thighs, removed his index finger from the patient's bottom and took the scissors from MacLeod.

'Thank you, Sir.'

The tie was cut and the student released. The student straightened up, his tie cut an inch from the knot, and he raised his clenched fist to his mouth and coughed. The patient remained in the foetal position, tie dangling from his tail. MacLeod and Jones were speechless.

'I guess that's it, Sir?'

'In a manner of speaking, it is it,' said Dr Jones.

'I think that'll be all that we want from you at the moment,' added MacLeod.

'Thanks very much.'

The student turned to the patient's bottom.

'You've been great,' he said addressing the cheeks. 'Just perfect.'

And in acknowledgement of perfection the cheeks clenched on the tie.

'Thank you very much,' said Dr Jones. 'You may go on to the next stage of the exam now. Thank you so much.'

'And thank you again,' Jones said to the bottom. 'Most kind, very helpful indeed. We're leaving the room now. Do feel free to relax. We'll be back shortly.'

And with that Jones ushered MacLeod out of the room following the medical student at a distance as he walked to the invigilation station.

'What do you think, Jones? Pass that one, too? Surely not?'

'I think we should, you know. The boy had great presence of mind and that bodes well for his future in medicine. An unequivocal pass with consideration given for honours.'

'What!?'

'Definitely. He's given us a story that we can tell and re-tell for the rest of our lives. Just think of it – when we're at that dinner table passing the port – MacLeod, he's given us a wonderful gift!

'And when we finish telling the story, they'll all ask whether or not we passed the boy. Can you imagine the laughter when we tell them that we did? MacLeod, we *have* to pass him. We've got to think about the dinner parties. It's a much better end to the story than telling them we failed the little bugger.'